Chronic Cardiac Disease

Optimizing Therapeutic Efficacy
in Heart Failure

Chronic Cardiac Disease

Optimizing Therapeutic Efficacy in Heart Failure

SIMON STEWART RN, PhD, NFESC, FAHA

National Heart Foundation of Australia/Roche Chair of Cardiovascular Nursing,
School of Nursing and Midwifery, University of South Australia
and
Clinical Research Initiative,
University of Glasgow, Scotland

Consulting Editor in Nursing

BRIAN DOLAN

W

WHURR PUBLISHERS
LONDON AND PHILADELPHIA

© 2002 Whurr Publishers

Whurr Publishers Ltd
19b Compton Terrace, London N1 2UN, England and
325 Chestnut Street, Philadelphia PA19106, USA

British Library Cataloguing in Publication Data

A catalogue record for this book is available from the
British Library.

ISBN 1 86156 290 X

Printed and bound in the UK by Athenaeum Press
Limited, Gateshead, Tyne & Wear.

Contents

Preface

The general public's view of heart disease is that of the 1960s stereotype; middle-aged men suffering a myocardial infarction, with dramatic symptoms, frantic therapeutic effort and frequently fatal outcome. We can now reflect that this scenario has become the exception, rather than the rule! Data from nearly all developed countries demonstrate that the age-adjusted incidence of myocardial infarction and of cardiac death is falling, although this fall is less clear-cut in lower socioeconomic groups.

It is superficially surprising, therefore, that what has emerged from recent evaluations is that the prevalence of heart disease in most communities is rising steadily, and that this is reflected on costs of hospitalization, if not in mortality data. It can be considered that most of the strategies directed at reducing risk, of ischaemic heart disease (such as cessation of smoking or cholesterol lowering) should be regarded as means of postponing disease onset rather than as 'vaccines' against eventual ischaemia. Improved survival rates for patients with acute myocardial infarction with therapy such as thrombolytic agents, coronary angio-plasty, beta-blockers and ACE inhibitors also leave more individuals susceptible to chronic heart disease and have contributed to the modern-day epidemic that heart failure represents.

This book describes recent research examining the overall burden and prognostic impact of heart failure in the United Kingdom. It is within this context that it also describes recent research that shows how it is possible to minimize the impact of heart failure through specialist nurse management of this complex syndrome. As the latter research was undertaken in Australia, it is especially important to note that this book also provides evidence to suggest that heart failure programmes developed in Australia are relevant to other developed countries. As such, heart failure does not respect arbitrary boundaries and truly represents an international epidemic.

Simon Stewart

Acknowledgements

This book represents a 'tale of two cities' – Adelaide, Australia and Glasgow, Scotland. The studies examining the role of specialist nurse interventions were undertaken as part of my PhD studies at the University of Adelaide, whereas the studies examining the current burden of heart failure were undertaken as part of my post-doctoral fellowship, at the University of Glasgow. I have been more than fortunate to have the friendship and guidance of two great men – Professor John Horowitz in Adelaide, and Professor John McMurray in Glasgow. I can only add my own humble sentiments of respect and awe at their achievements in the field of cardiovascular medicine and count myself extremely lucky that they have chosen to offer me their friendship and guidance. Likewise, I am eternally grateful to the continued support of the National Heart Foundation of Australia, which has funded both my PhD and post-doctoral research.

Lastly, I would like to dedicate this book to my wife Tania and my three beautiful daughters Laura, Amy and Sarah. I would be lost without all four of you and could never have completed any of these projects without your continued love and support.

CHAPTER 1

Heart failure: A modern epidemic we had to have?

Introduction

Cardiovascular disease, in particular coronary artery disease, continues to be the number one cause of premature death throughout western developed countries while consuming a considerable proportion of healthcare resources.[1] For example, a recent analysis of data from the Framingham Study suggests that the lifetime risk of developing coronary artery disease at the age of 40 is one in two for men and one in three for women.[2]

Although impressive moves have been made to curb the incidence of coronary artery disease in the past few decades, especially among individuals aged less than 75 years, the trend towards larger and significantly older populations in western developed countries[3, 4] together with better overall treatment of coronary artery disease among younger people has meant that its prevalence has increased markedly among older individuals.[1] For example, data for the period 1987–94 in the United States suggested that although the annual rate of hospitalization for acute myocardial infarction (AMI) was stable (representing about two and four hospitalizations/1000 women and men respectively), the survival rate following an admission for AMI was markedly increased.[5] The observed improvement in survival rates related to AMI has been confirmed by recent data from Scotland for 1986–95.[6] These data also showed that people who had experienced a first-ever AMI are becoming progressively older.[6]

The burden of coronary artery disease in the twenty-first century

The characteristics and impact of coronary artery disease in Australia over the past few decades are a good example of worldwide trends.[1] For example, the National Heart Foundation of Australia has reported about a 50% reduction in age-adjusted cardiovascular mortality over the past 20–30 years in Australia.[7] However, in 1994, 43% of all deaths in Australia were still attributable to cardiovascular disease; coronary artery disease was the largest single cause of death, accounting for 25% of deaths.[7] In this respect, Australia compares favourably with some northern European countries and has similar rates and trends to those reported in the United States, but compares poorly with other countries (most notably France and Japan).[7, 8]

The treatment-response paradox

The major advance in treating coronary artery disease has been the considerable reduction in the number of 'premature deaths' associated with the condition (defined as any death occurring five years or more below the average lifespan).[7, 8] This is not surprising considering the combined impact of more effective primary prevention, acute treatment and secondary prevention strategies designed to reduce the overall incidence of the common risk factors of coronary artery disease (thereby minimizing the risk of its development), to improve the immediate survival prospects for individuals who do have an acute coronary event and to modify their risk profile and longer-term survival prospects thereafter. Such strategies include:

1. Implementation of large-scale anti-smoking and exercise campaigns designed to combat smoking, sedentary lifestyles and obesity.[7]
2. Introduction of more effective lipid-lowering agents and identification of more effective targets for reducing cholesterol levels; in particular, low density lipoprotein cholesterol. In this respect a number of recent studies, including the 4S,[9] WOSCOPS,[10] CARE[11] and LIPID Study[12] have shown that aggressive lowering of cholesterol levels with 3-hydroxy-3-methylglutaryl coenzyme A reductase inhibitors (for example, simvastatin and pravastatin) is effective in both primary and secondary prevention. For example, in the 4S study of individuals with known coronary heart disease and hypercholesterolaemia, treatment with simvastatin was associated with a 30% reduction in mortality during follow-up compared with patients in the control group.[9]
3. Introduction of more effective anti-hypertensive agents and identification of more effective targets for lowering systolic and diastolic blood pressures in hypertensive individuals. For example, the recent HOT Study[13] showed that more intensive lowering of blood pressure in hypertensive individuals (aiming for a target diastolic pressure of 80 mm Hg using the long-acting calcium channel antagonist felodipine either with or without an angiotensin-converting enzyme (ACE) inhibitor or a β-adrenoceptor blocker) was associated with a lower rate of cardiovascular events.[13]
4. Introduction of more effective treatment strategies for the immediate management of acute coronary syndromes, including thrombolytics [14-17] and/or primary percutaneous angioplasty[18-21] in the management of an evolving AMI, in addition to use of ACE inhibitors to prevent late deterioration of ventricular function post AMI.[22-3]

5. Introduction of more effective treatment (the most notable being ACE inhibitors[24-7]) of chronic asymptomatic and symptomatic heart failure resulting in more prolonged survival among such patients.[28, 29]

Paradoxically, however, the initially improved survival prospects of individuals with AMI[5, 6, 30] have contributed to a population of older patients who are more susceptible to morbidity associated with advanced coronary artery disease and/or the development of chronic heart failure.[29, 31] As Kelly (1997) appropriately warns, our apparent ability to reduce the incidence of coronary artery disease (even when taking into account the common practice of ignoring the subsequent 'age creep' of coronary artery disease into much older, and less scrutinized, age groups) is being undermined by larger populations, and therefore by its increasing prevalence. The problems associated with a greater prevalence of older individuals with coronary artery disease (representing the 'residual' effects of better health strategies overall) are becoming increasingly apparent – for example, the increasing burden of chronic heart failure on healthcare systems throughout western developed countries.[1]

Other residual issues of coronary artery disease prevention and treatment

As with most treatment strategies, however, the advances in primary and secondary intervention are far from perfect, although they do contribute to the changing pattern of coronary artery disease. In Australia, the risk factor profile for coronary artery disease of the population remains unacceptably high – for example, recent estimates suggest that even in a relatively healthy population (as in Australia) about 15% of people need active treatment for hypertension (not counting the significant proportion of the population who are hypertensive but who have not been detected as such) and almost a quarter are active smokers.[7] These data suggest that coronary artery disease will continue to be associated with high rates of premature morbidity and mortality for the foreseeable future. Similarly, it is well known that proven pharmacological strategies including thrombolytic treatment for AMI[32] and the use of ACE inhibitors to prevent and treat heart failure[33-5] are frequently underused. This situation also applies to non-pharmacological strategies – for example, it is estimated that less than half of the patients with coronary artery disease in Europe and the United States receive appropriate cardiac rehabilitation.[28]

The combined failure of primary and secondary prevention measures

Clearly, therefore, there are two major problems confronting western developed countries in limiting the future impact of cardiovascular disease and in particular coronary artery disease. The first of these is the considerable proportion of individuals in the population (particularly in lower socioeconomic groups) who do not embrace or adhere to primary prevention strategies and who therefore have an increased risk of developing symptomatic coronary artery disease. The second problem relates to the increasing number of patients who survive a first ischaemic event (for example, an AMI) and are therefore likely to develop more acute ischaemic events thereafter, or who require chronic management for chronic angina pectoris or chronic heart failure, especially if secondary prevention strategies are incomplete by virtue of inadequate prescribed measures and/or poor compliance.

The cost of health care associated with coronary artery disease

The cost of managing cardiovascular disease is enormous. For example, $A3.5 billion (about £1.2 billion) is a conservative estimate of the cost of managing cardiovascular disease in Australia (representing a relatively small population of less than 20 million people.[7] A major component of this expenditure is hospital admissions. In 1994 there were about 20,000 admissions associated with AMI; male patients accounted for two-thirds of such hospitalizations and three-quarters had a 'first presentation' MI.[7] Statistics from 1995–6 indicate that circulatory disorders were the leading cause of public hospital admissions for an illness (almost 300,000 admissions in total) and resulted in 1.6 million days of hospitalization in public hospitals (second only to disorders of the nervous system) in Australia. Reports from other western developed countries indicate the huge costs associated with the most common manifestations of cardiovascular disease. For example, data from the United States suggest that the total combined costs of AMI and stroke in that country amount to nearly $US500,000 per second.[36] Consistent with data from Canada[37] and Finland[38], Jonsson reported that the management of cardiovascular disease states consumes almost 15% of annual healthcare expenditure in Sweden.[39]

Summary

The general public's view of coronary heart disease is that of the 1960s stereotype; middle-aged male patients suffering cardiac emergencies such as myocardial infarction, with dramatic symptoms, frantic therapeutic effort and frequently fatal outcome. We can now reflect that this scenario has become the exception rather than the rule: the age-adjusted incidence of myocardial infarction and of cardiac death is falling in most western countries[8], although this fall is less clear-cut in lower socioeconomic groups.[40, 41]

It is superficially surprising, therefore, that what has emerged from recent evaluations is that the *prevalence* of heart disease in most communities is rising steadily, and that this is reflected in the costs of hospitalization, if not in mortality data. Most of the strategies directed at reducing the risk of ischaemic heart disease (such as stopping smoking or lowering cholesterol) should be regarded as means of postponing the onset of disease rather than as 'vaccines' against eventual ischaemia. Improved survival rates for patients with acute myocardial infarction with treatment such as thrombolytic agents[14], coronary angioplasty[19] and ACE inhibitors[22] also mean that more individuals have chronic heart disease (most notably chronic heart failure[42]), and in elderly people increasing rates of atrial fibrillation[43] and aortic stenosis[44] contribute to the complexity and overall burden imposed by cardiac disability.

The major stimulus to the diagnosis of chronic heart failure is the institution of appropriate *treatment*. It is in this regard that recent reports (for example, the CASE Study in Australia[45]) are most revealing.[33, 34] There have been dramatic advances in the management of chronic heart failure in the past 15 years, resulting in considerable improvement in outcomes for this patient population[29] – although there is clearly greater scope for further reductions in both morbidity[42] and mortality.[46] ACE inhibitors (preferably in the largest tolerated dose), [47] spironolactone[48] and β-adrenoceptor antagonists[49] have all been shown to reduce mortality and morbidity in patients with left ventricular systolic dysfunction; there is also evidence supporting the use of angiotensin receptor antagonists or hydralazine/ nitrates in patients intolerant to ACE inhibitors.

It is therefore an important finding of a recent study in Australia (even in the hands of an 'interested' cohort of general practitioners) that patients with chronic heart failure were treated with ACE inhibitors in little more than half of the cases, usually with low dose regimens. Relative to this, the use of diuretics and digoxin was surprisingly high when current recommendations were considered. This makes it clear that chronic heart failure is largely under-treated in Australia, [45] as it is in many other developed countries. [33-5] The price to pay, of course, is increased risk of deterioration, hospitalization and death.

The epidemic of chronic heart failure in elderly people has its counterpart in an explosion of recent relevant clinical trial information. The HOPE Study results suggest that all patients at high risk of ischaemia should be considered for treatment with ACE inhibitors, irrespective of the presence or absence of chronic heart failure.[50] The data on the beneficial effect of spironolactone[48] and some of the β-adrenoceptor antagonist data are quite recent.[49]

It is in this context that the identification of optimal treatment and management protocols for these patients constitutes a major challenge for the new millennium. Before discussing how best this can be achieved, the following chapters provide a comprehensive overview of the causes and pharmacological treatment of heart failure, in addition to recent estimates of the current burden imposed by heart failure in the UK.

References

1.   Kelly D. Our future society: A global challenge. *Circulation* 1997; 95: 2459–64.
2.   Lloyd-Jones D, Larson M, Beiser A, et al. Lifetime risk of developing coronary heart disease. *Lancet* 1999; 353: 89–92.

3.   *World Population Projections*. Baltimore, MD: John Hopkins University Press, 1990.

4.   Caselli G, Lopez A. *Health and Mortality among Elderly Populations*. New York, NY: Clarendon Press, 1996.

5.   Rosamond W, Chambless L, Folsom A, et al. Trends in the incidence of myocardial infarction and in mortality due to coronary heart disease, 1987 to 1994. *N Engl J Med* 1998; 339: 861–7.

6.   Capewell S, Livingstone BM, MacIntyre K, et al. Trends in case-fatality in 117, 718 patients admitted with acute myocardial infarction in Scotland. *Eur Heart J* 2001; 21: 1833–40.

7.   Heart Foundation of Australia. *Heart and Stroke Facts*. Canberra: Heart Foundation of Australia, 1996.

8.   Tunstall-Pedoe H, Kuulasmaa K, Mahonen M, et al. Contribution of trends in survival and coronary-event rates to changes in coronary heart disease mortality: 10 year results from 37 WHO MONICA Project populations. *Lancet* 1999; 353: 1547–57.

9.   Scandinavian Simvastatin Survival Study Group. Randomised trial of cholesterol lowering in 4444 patients with coronary heart disease: The Scandinavian Simvastatin Survival Study (4S). *Lancet* 1994; 344: 1383–9.

10.   Sheperd J, Cobbe S, Ford I, et al., for the West of Scotland Coronary Prevention Study Group. Prevention of coronary heart disease with pravastatin in men with hypercholesterolaemia. *N Engl J Med* 1995; 333: 1301–7.

11.   Sacks F, Pfeffer M, Moye LA, et al., for the Cholesterol and Recurrent Events Trial Investigators. The effect of pravastatin on coronary events after myocardial infarction in patients with average cholesterol levels. *N Engl J Med* 1996; 335: 1001–9.

12.   The LIPID Study Group. Prevention of cardiovascular events and death with pravastatin in patients with coronary heart disease and a broad range of initial cholesterol levels. The Long-Term Intervention with Pravastatin in Ischaemic Disease (LIPID) Study Group. *N Engl J Med* 1998; 339: 1349–57.

13.   Hansson L, Zanchetti A, Carruthers S, et al., for the HOT Study Group. Effects of intensive blood-pressure lowering and low-dose aspirin in patients with hypertension: Principal results of the Hypertension Optimal Treatment (HOT) trial. *Lancet* 1998; 351: 1755–62.

14.   The GISSI Investigators. Effectiveness of intravenous thrombolytic treatment in acute myocardial infarction. *Lancet* 1986; 327: 397–401.

15.   The ISIS-2 Investigators. Randomised trial of intravenous streptokinase, oral aspirin, both or neither among 17, 187 cases of suspected acute myocardial infarction: ISIS-2. *Lancet* 1988; 332: 349–59.

16.   The GISSI-2 Investigators. A factorial randomised trial of alteplase versus streptokinase and heparin versus no heparin among 12, 490 patients with acute myocardial infarction. *Lancet* 1990; 336: 65–71.

17.   The ISIS-3 Investigators. A randomised comparison of streptokinase vs tissue plasminogen activator versus antistreplase and of aspirin plus heparin vs aspirin alone among 41, 299 cases of suspected acute myocardial infarction. *Lancet* 1992; 339: 753–70.

18.   The GUSTO Investigators. An international randomised trial comparing four thrombolytic strategies for acute myocardial infarction. *N Engl J Med* 1993; 329: 673–82.

19.   The PAMI Trial Investigators. Analysis of the relative costs and effectiveness of primary angioplasty versus tissue-type plasminogen activator: The Primary Angioplasty in Myocardial Infarction (PAMI) trial. *J Am Coll Cardiol* 1997; 29: 901–7.

20.   The Myocardial Infarction Triage and Intervention Investigators. A comparison of thrombolytic therapy with primary coronary angioplasty for acute myocardial infarction. *N Engl J Med* 1996; 335: 1253–60.

21. The GUSTO IIb Angioplasty Substudy Investigators. A clinical trial comparing primary coronary angioplasty with tissue plasminogen activator for acute myocardial infarction. *N Engl J Med* 1997; 336: 1621–8.

22. Rutherford J, Pfeffer M, Moye LA, et al. Effects of captopril on ischemic events after myocardial infarction. Results of the Survival and Ventricular Enlargement (SAVE) Trial. *Circulation* 1994; 90: 1731–8.

23. Pfeffer M, Braunwald E, Moye LA, et al. Effect of captopril on mortality and morbidity in patients with left ventricular dysfunction after myocardial infarction: Results of the Survival and Ventricular Enlargement Trial. *N Engl J Med* 1992; 327: 669–77.

24. The Captopril Multicenter Research Group. A placebo-controlled trial of captopril in refractory chronic congestive heart failure. *J Am Coll Cardiol* 1983; 2: 755–63.

25. The CONSENSUS Trial Study Group. Effects of enalapril on mortality in severe congestive heart failure: Results of the Cooperative North Scandinavian Enalapril Survival Study (CONSENSUS). *N Engl J Med* 1987; 316: 1429–35.

26. The SOLVD Investigators. Effect of enalapril on survival in patients with reduced left ventricular ejection fractions and congestive heart failure. *N Engl J Med* 1991; 325: 293–302.

27. The SOLVD Investigators. Effect of enalapril on mortality and the development of heart failure in asymptomatic patients with reduced left ventricular ejection fractions. *N Engl J Med* 1992; 327: 685–91.

28. Wood D, for the EUROASPIRE Study Group. EUROASPIRE – A European Society of Cardiology survey of secondary prevention of coronary heart disease: Principal results. *Eur Heart J* 1997; 18: 1569–82.

29. Pearson T, McBride P, Miller N, et al. Organization of preventative cardiology service (Task Force 8 of the 27th Bethesda Conference). *J Am Coll Cardiol* 1996; 27: 1039–47.

30. Abrahamsson P, Dellborg M, Rosengren A, et al. Improved long term prognosis after myocardial infarction 1984–1991. *Eur Heart J* 1998; 19: 1512–17.

31. Kannel W. Epidemiology and prevention of cardiac failure: Framingham Study insights. *Eur Heart J* 1987; 8 (Supp F): 23–9.

32. McLaughlin T, Soumerari S, Willison D, et al. Adherence to national guidelines for drug treatment of suspected acute myocardial infarction: Evidence for undertreatment in women and the elderly. *Arch Intern Med* 1996; 156: 799–805.

33. Edep ME, Shah NB, Tateo IM, et al. Difference between primary care physicians and cardiologists in management of congestive heart failure: Relation to practice guidelines. *J Am Coll Cardiol* 1997; 30: 518–26.

34. Ghali J, Giles T, Gonzales M, et al. Patterns of physician use of angiotensin converting enzyme inhibitors in the inpatient treatment of congestive heart failure. *J La State Med Soc* 1997; 149: 474–84.

35. Luzier A, Forrest A, Adelman M, et al. Impact of angiotensin-converting enzyme inhibitor underdosing on rehospitalization rates in congestive heart failure. *Am J Cardiol* 1998; 82: 465–9.

36. Egan B, Lackland D. Strategies for cardiovascular disease prevention: Importance of public and community health programs. *Ethnicity Dis* 1998; 8: 228–39.

37. Chan B, Coyte P, Heick C. Economic impact of cardiovascular disease in Canada. *Can J Cardiol* 1996; 12: 1000–6.

38. Kiiskinen U, Vartianinen E, Pekurinen M, et al. Does prevention of cardiovascular disease lead to decreased cost of illness? Twenty years of experience from Finland. *Prev Med* 1997; 26: 220–6.

39. Jonsson B. Measurement of health outcome and associated costs in cardiovascular disease. *Eur Heart J* 1996; 17 (suppl): A2–A7.

40. Morrison C, Woodward M, Leslie W, et al. Effect of socio-economic group on the incidence of, management of, and survival after myocardial infarction and coronary death: Analysis of community coronary event register. *BMJ* 1997; 314: 541–6.

41. MacIntyre K, Stewart S, Chalmers S, et al. Relation between socioeconomic deprivation and death from a first acute myocardial infarction in Scotland: Population based analysis. *BMJ* 2001; 322: 1152–3.

42. Stewart S, MacIntyre K, McCleod MC, et al. Trends in heart failure hospitalisations in Scotland, 1990–1996: An epidemic that has reached its peak? *Eur Heart J* 2000; 22: 209–17.

43. Stewart S, MacIntyre K, McCleod ME, et al. Trends in hospital activity, morbidity and case fatality related to atrial fibrillation in Scotland, 1986–96. *Eur Heart J* 2001; 22: 693–701

44. Unger SA, Robinson MA, Horowitz JD. Perhexiline improves symptomatic status in elderly patients with severe aortic stenosis. *Aust NZ J Med* 1997; 27: 24–8.

45. Krum H, Tonkin AM, Currie R, et al. Chronic heart failure in Australian general practice. The Cardiac Awareness Survey and Evaluation (CASE) Study. *MJA* 2001; 174: 439–44.

46. Stewart S, MacIntyre K, Hole DA, et al. More malignant than cancer? Five-year survival following a first admission for heart failure in Scotland? *Eur J Heart Fail* 2001; 3: 315–22.

47. Packer M, Poole-Wilson PA, Armstrong PW, et al. Comparative effects of low and high doses of the angiotensin converting enzyme inhibitor, lisinopril, on morbidity and mortality in chronic heart failure. *Circulation* 1999; 100: 2312–18.

48. Pitt B, Zannad F, Remme WJ, et al. The effect of spironolactone on morbidity and mortality in patients with severe heart failure. Randomized Aldactone Evaluation Study Investigators. *N Engl J Med* 1999; 341: 709–17.

49. MERIT Investigators. Effect of metoprolol CR/XL in chronic heart failure: Metoprolol CR/XL Randomised Intervention Trial in Congestive Heart Failure (Merit-HF). *Lancet* 1999; 353: 2001–7.

50. Yusuf S, Sleight P, Pogue J, et al. Effects of an angiotensin-converting enzyme inhibitor, ramipril, on cardiovascular events in high-risk patients. The Heart Outcomes Prevention Evaluation Study Investigators. *N Engl J Med* 2000; 342: 145–53.

CHAPTER 2

Clinical characteristics and management of chronic heart failure: Future implications

Introduction

As discussed in Chapter 1, the combination of increased survival following acute myocardial infarction (AMI) and generally older patient populations will most probably result in an increased prevalence of chronic disease states such as chronic heart failure, with recent evidence suggesting that heart failure is likely to become the cardiac 'epidemic' of the new millennium.[1] This chapter represents an overview of the pathophysiology, treatment, incidence, prevalence and associated burden of chronic heart failure, with particular emphasis on the issues that affect the management and subsequent health outcomes of the subset of individuals with heart failure who develop severe congestive heart failure and who remain symptomatic despite conventional therapy.

Clinical definition and characteristics of chronic heart failure

Congestive heart failure represents a complex pathological process and is associated with a broad spectrum of clinical presentations, thereby defying simple explanation and definition.[2] For the purpose of this discussion, however, the term chronic heart failure will be frequently used in the context of its most common manifestation – chronic congestive heart failure. As such, Packer (1992) defines chronic congestive heart failure as: 'a complex syndrome characterized by abnormalities of left ventricular function and neurohormonal regulation which are accompanied by effort intolerance, fluid retention and reduced longevity'.[3]

This definition includes the two of the most distinctive components of congestive heart failure – the underlying pathology of ventricular dysfunction (whether it be primarily systolic or diastolic) and the typical, clinical presentation of patients with this syndrome. This does not presuppose, however, that left ventricular dysfunction will automatically manifest itself in a consistent symptomatic and clinical form. In fact there is usually a poor correlation between the clinical parameters of failure (for example, left ventricular ejection fraction) and the patient's functional status.[4] One of the major reasons for poor correlation between degree of impairment of systolic function and symptomatic status is the variable extent of diastolic ventricular interaction, a phenomenon that is difficult to detect clinically.[5, 6] In general, however, chronic congestive heart failure secondary to reduced systolic function is accepted as being a syndrome in which the heart is unable to deliver enough blood to meet the body's metabolic demands and, if this 'mismatch' is severe enough, an individual with chronic heart failure will typically experience symptoms of breathlessness, fatigue and fluid congestion.[7]

Pathophysiology of chronic heart failure

The current paradigm of the pathogenesis and subsequent treatment of chronic heart failure assumes that, regardless of the initial stimuli (whether it be AMI, chronic valvular disease and/or prolonged hypertension), its development reflects the longer-term failure and subsequent adverse effects of adaptive changes to the structure and stimulation of the heart that were initially triggered to maintain an adequate cardiac output.[3] The two principal components in this maladaptive process are ventricular remodelling and neuroendocrine activation. What follows is an overview of the current understanding of the pathology that contributes to the development of left ventricular systolic dysfunction and the clinical syndrome of chronic heart failure.

Initial myocardial injury

Chronic heart failure is most often associated with the development of ischaemic cardiomyopathy following an AMI, affecting a localized area of the left ventricle and with associated loss of left ventricular systolic function.[8] However, non-ischaemic heart failure is also common, with genetic, post-viral, drug-induced congestive cardiomyopathy and hypertensive, congenital and valvular disease being possible causes.[9–11]

The initial response to myocardial injury

Regardless of the cause, there is a critical loss of functioning myocardial cells, and the heart's inability to adequately empty the ventricle (for example, because of localized paradoxical wall motion of the left anterior ventricular wall following an AMI) during systole increases diastolic pressure (preload). With the associated loss of cardiac output typically resulting in hypo-perfusion of the kidney, the renin-angiotensin system is activated, releasing both angiotensin II (a potent vasoconstrictor) and aldosterone (which increases sodium retention), both of which increase cardiac preload and therefore the left ventricular end-diastolic volume. Moreover, the reduced cardiac output results in increased stimulation of the baroreceptors, leading to sympathetic activation and stimulation of β-adrenergic receptors in the non-injured myocardium, and both the force and the frequency of ventricular contractions increase.[12] There is also progressive impairment of the myocardial force-frequency relationship, resulting in accentuation of symptoms during tachycardia.[13, 14]

This initial adaptive response puts greater stress on the left ventricular wall during diastole and is only a short-term solution.[15] As part of the longer-term response, the heart undergoes a structural change in order to reduce ventricular wall stress while optimizing cardiac output. This phenomenon is known as 'ventricular remodelling'.

Ventricular remodelling

This process represents the structural changes that occur in ventricular chamber size, wall thickness and composition.[16] In accordance with Laplace's Law (T = P × r/2h, where T is tension, P is pressure and h is wall thickness), in order to maintain wall tension and improve cardiac efficiency, an increased synthesis of myofibrillar proteins produces greater wall thickness (left ventricular hypertrophy).[17] This change occurs because the only pathway for ventricular enlargement is through hypertrophy of pre-existing myocytes rather than the regeneration or replacement of those damaged by the initial injury (for example, an AMI).[18, 19] To support this structural change there is a parallel increase in myocardial collagen content; [20] Beltrami et al. (1995) showed that in end-stage ischaemic cardiomyopathy, the extent of interstitial fibrosis was frequently disproportionate to the original myocardial injury.[21]

Although the exact stimulus and mechanism for myocardial hypertrophy is not completely understood, it is clear that mechanical (for example, the direct stress of increased preload and associated chamber dilatation) and neuroendocrine factors are involved. For example, ventricular remodelling in animal models has been stimulated by the presence of norepinephrine, atrial natriuretic factor, arginine vasopressin and angiotensin II.[22-4] In this context it is clear that the process of ventricular remodelling is a dynamic one, especially among individuals with severe heart failure.[25, 26]

If the process of remodelling is not sufficient to maintain wall tension the individual will begin to experience symptoms secondary to the subsequent ventricular dysfunction and limited cardiac output, especially as this is associated with further ventricular dilatation and possibly further myocyte loss. The shape and size of the 'remodelled' ventricle either with or without left ventricular chamber dilatation will vary according to the type and severity of myocardial injury and the character of stress (for example, increased preload and possibly afterload, extent of myocyte loss/contractility).[27] For example, concentric hypertrophy is frequently associated with prolonged cardiovascular stress secondary to chronic hypertension or valvular disease, affecting the left ventricle as a whole.[12]

Sustained neuroendocrine activation

When the systemic perfusion pressure falls secondary to the lower cardiac output associated with myocardial injury, two initial mechanisms reflecting a neuroendocrine response are activated: peripheral vasoconstriction and sodium retention. As discussed above, the initial vasoconstriction and sodium retention associated with chronic heart failure reflect enhanced sympathetic activation and activation of the renin-angiotensin system designed to increase cardiac preload and consequently cardiac output. However, in the longer term it seems that each hormonal system plays a role in maintaining vasoconstriction in some patients.[28] Moreover, a number of locally acting vasoconstrictors produced by the endothelium are more active in chronic heart failure. For example, concentrations of endothelin have been shown to increase in proportion to the severity of heart failure.[29] There is also some evidence that tissue responses to endothelial-derived relaxing factor, which normally counterbalances the influence of endothelin, [30] and atrial natriuretic peptide (despite elevated levels), which normally inhibits release of noradrenaline, renin and vasopressin, [31, 32] are attenuated in chronic heart failure. The beneficial effects of local prostanoid secretion are therefore critical, and susceptible to inhibition if cyclo-oxygenase inhibitors are co-prescribed.[33, 34]

Like the mechanical changes described above, although enhanced neuroendocrine activation can initially be beneficial, it can cause paradoxical worsening of cardiac function and emergence of severe symptoms characteristic of congestive heart failure.

Role of oncogene activation

The deterioration in ventricular function, as described above, is not purely a result of changes in afterload or of the heart 'giving up'. Other cellular processes contribute to heart failure following an initial myocardial injury. For example, the role of apoptosis in the pathology of myocyte loss and development of advanced heart failure has been the subject of considerable interest. The genes involved in apoptosis, such as p53, have been shown to be regulated upwards in the failing canine heart.[35] Moreover, cytokines, such as TNF-α produced by activated macrophages, have been shown to induce apoptosis in model systems.[9] In this respect, elevated levels of TNF-α in chronic heart failure are associated with reduced cardiac contractility and a poorer overall prognosis.[36, 37]

The transition to clinically overt heart failure

Epidemiological data suggesting that a considerable proportion of patients with pathological changes indicative of ventricular remodelling remain functional without overt symptoms of heart failure[38] supports the proposition that the adaptive changes described above are frequently successful in maintaining an adequate cardiac output. Clearly, there is often a lengthy hiatus between the changes described above and the emergence of symptomatic heart failure.[3, 12] As such, it seems that overt symptoms of chronic heart failure will most likely occur when the adaptive process described above is overwhelmed by too great a myocardial injury (for example, after recurrent AMI) and/or the normal deterioration associated with advancing age.[16] As discussed above, there is no consistent correlation between the commonly measured parameters of ventricular dysfunction (for example, left ventricular ejection fraction) and an individual's symptomatic profile.[4] However, there is clearly a subset of individuals in the total population of patients with chronic heart failure in whom left ventricular dysfunction and severe symptoms of congestion and functional impairment are evident. In a review of the relevant literature Adams and Zannard (1998) suggest that individuals with severe congestive heart failure can typically identified on the following basis:

1. Persistence of severe clinical signs and symptoms of heart failure despite treatment.
2. Marked left ventricular systolic dysfunction.
3. Poor exercise capacity.

As such, these individuals (as will be discussed in the following chapter) are far more likely to suffer significant morbidity and to die prematurely.[39]

Pathological and clinical characteristics of severe chronic congestive heart failure

Apart from the fact that the normal adaptive and protective responses to the potential loss of cardiac output resulting from myocardial injury have probably failed in individuals with severe chronic congestive heart failure, what differentiates them from most individuals with chronic heart failure who are clinically stable? This section gives an overview of some of the important pathological and clinical characteristics of severe congestive heart failure, once again with particular emphasis on those patients with associated ischaemic cardiomyopathy and impaired left ventricular systolic function.

Left ventricular hypertrophy

Patients with severe, congestive heart failure often have an enlarged left ventricle, secondary to the process of ventricular modelling described above. At rest, this adaptation may be associated with ventricular function that is almost normal, but during periods of exercise a marked elevation in pulmonary pressure (and therefore the development of pulmonary congestion) may occur without a sufficient increase in cardiac output.[40] The absence of rales and X-ray evidence of pulmonary congestion in patients assessed in a resting state is frequently misinterpreted as an indication of the absence of left-side heart failure and the presence of congestion.[41, 42] The persistent constraints on 'forward' cardiac output associated with inadequate adaptation of the left ventricular wall are also frequently associated with symptoms indicative of orthopnea and parox-ysmal nocturnal dyspnoea secondary to the increased preload associated with positional change, with the potential for development of acute pulmonary oedema.[43] Alternatively, peripheral oedema occurs in only about 25% of patients with severe heart failure and is more likely in the presence of concurrent pulmonary hypertension[43] and/or diastolic ventricular interaction.[5, 6] In this context, a number of studies have shown that the more spherical the left ventricle, the greater the depression of cardiac contractility, heart failure symptoms and risk of premature mortality.[44, 45]

Sudden death

Sudden death among patients with severe, advanced heart failure has been estimated to account for 28–68% of total mortality among those individuals being treated with an angiotensin-converting enzyme (ACE) inhibitor; [46, 47] most of these deaths are presumed to be secondary to a ventricular arrhythmia. Those patients with concurrent coronary heart disease may be at particular risk of fatal arrhythmic events.[48] A number of mechanisms may contribute to the genesis of ventricular arrhythmias in this clinical setting, including micro re-entry circuits in the vicinity of large infarction scars, [49] the presence of interstitial fibrosis and abnormal intracellular calcium handling, [48] elevated sympathetic tone, [50] and depletion of magnesium and potassium.[51]

Chronic myocardial ischaemia/'hibernation'

Patients with severe heart failure are also at risk of chronic sub-endocardial ischaemia, in some cases leading to a vicious circle of further dysfunction of the left ventricle.[9] The sub-endocardium of a dilated ventricle is particularly vulnerable to ischaemia secondary to the combination of increased wall stress and increased oxygen requirements.[52] Any factor that limits coronary perfusion (for example, coronary heart disease, tachycardia or increased diastolic filling pressures[53]) is likely to affect the sub-endocardium first.[54] As such, sub-endocardial ischaemia is not confined to patients with ischaemic cardiomyopathy, and individuals with primary cardiomyopathy have also been shown to experience such ischaemia, which may occur in the absence of pain.[55] A different potential adaptation to chronic reduction in the availability of high-energy phosphates is reduced contrac-tility of viable myocardium resulting in ablution of both contraction and ischaemia. This is termed myocardial hibernation.[56, 57] Hibernation presents major diagnostic challenges in a prospective sense, and has been treated to date only through coronary revascularization.[58]

Progressive myocyte loss

Progressive myocyte loss secondary to necrosis or apoptosis seems to be another important pathological component of progressive left ventricular dysfunction.[59, 60] In a number of animal models exposure to cardiac norepinephrine, angiotensin II[61] and aldosterone[62, 63] has been shown to produce myocardial necrosis; of interest, considering the recent results of the RALES study examining the relative efficacy of spironolactone in this clinical setting (as will be discussed later)[64], was the fact that the deleterious effects of aldosterone in this respect were ameliorated by the addition of low-dose spironolactone.

Peripheral changes

In the longer term, as cardiac function declines, the redistribution of blood flow away from the peripheral circulation towards the vital organs through peripheral vasoconstriction is maintained, even in the basal state.[65, 66] As discussed above, factors such as depressed endothelium-dependent vasodilatation[67, 68] and increased endothelin levels of a pulmonary origin contribute to this phenomenon.[69] However, the reduction in peripheral blood flow does not seem to wholly explain the muscle loss and fatigue on exertion common to patients with severe heart failure[70, 71] and this remains the subject of much conjecture.[9] In severe heart failure the redistribution of blood flow away from the gastro-intestinal tract also contributes to anorexia and associated wasting. As such, cardiac cachexia has been reported to be present in up to 15% of patients with symptoms of severe heart failure.[72] Moreover, its presence has been correlated with increased morbidity and mortality.[73–5]

Peripheral vasoconstriction is also likely to disturb renal function: hence the role of the renin-angiotensin system. As such, many patients with severe heart failure frequently show elevated serum creatinine and liver enzymes, with a reduced serum sodium concentration being correlated with activation of the renin-angiotensin system[76] and compensatory prostanoid secretion.[33]

Acute deterioration

Clearly, patients with severe chronic congestive heart failure walk a tightrope between maintaining optimal cardiac function, becoming over-congested and developing acute pulmonary oedema. For example, a recent study suggested that the average patient hospitalized for decompensated heart failure undergoes more than 4L of net diuresis during the associated hospitalization.[77] In this context, there are a number of concurrent clinical factors that may adversely affect cardiac function further and therefore precipitate acute deterioration in such individuals. These include:

1. Acute myocardial ischaemia (for example, an acute coronary syndrome with or without new myocardial necrosis).

2. Arrhythmias (for example, atrial fibrillation, or bradyarrhythmia secondary to digoxin toxicity).
3. Uncontrolled and prolonged hypertension.
4. Worsening pulmonary disease (for example, respiratory infection in the presence of chronic airways limitation).
5. Deteriorating renal function (for example, secondary to progressive reno-vascular disease).[78, 79]

Incidence and prevalence of chronic heart failure

Because of the inherent difficulty in defining chronic heart failure overall and the fact that it is clear that the underlying pathophysiology of left ventricular dysfunction, whether it be primarily systolic or diastolic in nature, can be present without the emergence of clearly identifiable symptoms (for example, among individuals with undetected, chronic hypertension), there is a general lack of reliable epidemiological estimates of its prevalence, incidence and associated prognosis.[4] However, there is increasing recognition that the incidence and prevalence of chronic heart failure is likely to rise substantially in the immediate future.[1, 80] Moreover, a number of recent studies have attempted to address the lack of epidemiological data concerning chronic heart failure, albeit in generally younger populations than the predominantly older cohorts of hospitalized patients who present with severe congestive heart failure.[1]

For example, McDonagh and colleagues (1997) performed a cross-sectional survey of 1640 men and women aged 25–74 who participated in a MONICA coronary risk-factor survey undertaken in Glasgow, Scotland, in 1992 to determine the prevalence of left ventricular systolic dysfunction as determined by standard echocardiography. Overall, 2.9% of those screened were found to have a left ventricular fraction of ≤ 30%; almost half (1.4% of the total) being asymptomatic in this respect. Not surprisingly, most patients (83%) with left ventricular systolic dysfunction had evidence of ischaemic heart disease (as determined by electrocardiogram (ECG) criteria) compared with 21% of the remainder of the cohort. This was also true for the proportion of individuals in whom hypertension was also determined to be present, the corresponding figures being 72% vs 38%. Both of these differences were highly significant ($p < 0.001$). On multivariate analysis, angina (odds ratio 5.7), ECG evidence of ischaemia or MI (odds ratio 5.4), hypertension (odds ratio 2.4) and male gender (odds ratio 2.2) were all predictive of a left ventricular ejection fraction of < 30%. Of interest was the fact that 7.7% of individuals recorded a left ventricular ejection fraction of < 35%. Less surprising was the fact that the prevalence of left ventricular systolic dysfunction increased with age (among individuals aged 65–74 the prevalence was 6.4%) and there is little doubt that screening of an older cohort of individuals (those aged more than 72 years) would detect an even greater prevalence of this clinical entity.[38]

Importantly, the prevalence of symptomatic left ventricular systolic dysfunction in this particular cohort was similar to that reported in cohorts reflecting both the general population of the US[81] and that of the UK[82], although it was higher than that reported from the Framingham Study.[83, 84]

Overall, there are two types of studies of the incidence of chronic heart failure described in the literature – those that examine a population cohort at regular intervals to determine who has developed heart failure (for example, the Framingham Study in the US[85, 86] and the Study of Men Born in 1913 in Sweden[87]) and those that identify individuals who develop heart failure through a population-based surveillance system (for example, the Finnish Study, [88] the UK general practice survey[89] and the Dutch general practice surveys, [90, 91] the Rochester Study[92] and the US Two Counties Study[93]). As with studies examining the prevalence of heart failure, crude, unadjusted estimates of the incidence of heart failure in these studies vary markedly; ranging from 1.0 to 5.0 cases per 1000 population a year.[94] Most importantly, however, the incidence of heart failure rose markedly with age in all of these studies, with two of the most recent studies reporting an incidence rate as high as 40 cases per 1000 population a year among individuals aged 75 years and over.[89, 91]

The overall variability in terms of the definition, screening methods, target populations and coding of left ventricular dysfunction, with or without the clinical symptoms of heart failure, has led to markedly different estimations of the prevalence of chronic heart failure, and it renders nearly all of the studies undertaken in this respect of little value for projecting the overall prevalence of chronic heart failure to the overall population.[94]

Healthcare utilization and costs

Although the same inherent difficulties in estimating both the prevalence and incidence of chronic heart failure in the general population (for example, variability in defining and coding heart failure) also apply to hospital-based studies, such studies probably provide a more accurate reflection of the burden of heart failure to the healthcare system. For example, in the 1960s Klainer et al. (1966) reported that 1–2% of total admissions in selected hospitals in Australia, Canada and the United States were associated with overt heart failure.[95] More recently, a number of studies have shown that the rate of hospitalization for heart failure has been increasing steadily.[84, 96–104] For example, Ghali and colleagues (1990) examined rates of hospitalization for heart failure in the US during 1973–86.[84] During this period the number of admissions more than doubled. Of interest was the fact that the age-adjusted increase in admissions for heart failure was most pronounced among women, thereby equalizing the previous imbalance between men and women in 1978 and surpassing them thereafter in this regard. Among white women admissions for chronic heart failure resulted in 869 discharges per 100,000 in 1973, compared with 1633 discharges per 100,000 in 1986 – an increase of 88%. Over the same period white men had a 66% increase (in 1986 there were 1542 discharges per 100,000).[84] More recently, McMurray (1993) examined trends in hospitalization for heart failure in Scotland (comprising a relatively stable and well-characterized population of 5 million) for the period 1980–90.[99] It was found that during this period the rate of hospital admissions where heart failure was given as a primary diagnosis increased almost 60% from 1.3 to 2.1 admissions per 1000 population. This trend was also evident in the corresponding figures for hospital admissions associated with heart failure as either a primary or secondary diagnosis, with an increase from 2.5 to 4.2 admissions per 1000 population. Moreover, consistent with the US data from Ghali and colleagues that suggest that chronic heart failure is the leading cause of hospital admissions among individuals aged $\geq$ 65 years, [105–7] 78% of admissions occurred among individuals aged $\geq$ 68 years, and the number of men (48%) and women (52%) involved was about equal.

Not surprisingly, the cost of managing chronic heart failure is both enormous and rising. For example, in the early 1990s chronic heart failure was estimated to account for more than 5 million days of hospitalization and was a leading cause of cardiovascular-associated visits to primary care physicians, diagnostic procedures and prescribed medication in the US: associated healthcare expenditure was estimated to be in the order of $US8 billion a year.[106, 108] A parallel examination of the cost of heart failure to the National Health Service in the UK during the financial year 1990–1 by McMurray and colleagues (1993) revealed that the annual direct cost of heart failure was about £360 million, with hospitalization accounting for approximately 60% and prescribed medication only 8% of these costs. Overall, this represented 1% of the total National Health Service budget.[109]

Overall, the data from a large number of western developed countries consistently show that chronic heart failure puts a heavy burden on the incumbent healthcare system. Hospital admissions in particular represent the most costly component of this burden, consuming about two-thirds of the overall costs required to manage such patients.[110] Hospital admissions among patients with chronic heart failure are therefore a major contributor to estimated annual healthcare costs, equivalent to 1–2% of overall healthcare expenditure in developed counties.[98–102, 111–13] With the data showing that rates of hospitalization are continuing to rise, and that more than 400,000 people are diagnosed with chronic heart failure each year in the US, [114] it is not surprising that a more recent estimate of the cost of managing chronic heart failure in the US was upwards of $10 billion a year and rising.[115]

Pharmacological management of severe congestive heart failure

Management of chronic heart failure, and many other cardiac disease states, can be stratified into three principal components:

1. Prevention.
2. Limiting progression of the disease state if prevention fails.
3. Palliative alleviation of chronic symptoms.[116]

The current discussion will focus on limiting the progression of heart failure and the palliative management of those patients with severe congestive heart failure. Considering the relative cost of hospitalization compared with that of prescribed medication to total healthcare expenditure, [109] it is clear that the treatment strategies that include pharmacological agents that have the proven ability to limit hospital use over the lifespan of patients at risk of episodic bouts of acute heart failure requiring hospital admission will prove to be the most economically attractive.[117] Likewise, initially very expensive surgical procedures such as heart transplantation may prove to be cost-effective among younger individuals in terms of returned productivity, increased lifespan and reduced healthcare costs over a prolonged period. However, surgical options frequently have limited practical (or economic) value in the management of predominantly older patients with chronic congestive heart failure.[114] Long-term pharmacotherapy therefore represents the most common treatment option for this syndrome. Not surprisingly, however, considering the complex pathophysiology of chronic heart failure, patients with severe signs and symptoms of congestive heart failure frequently receive a complex cocktail of pharmacological agents that need constant adjustment to maintain clinical equilibrium (usually through physician consultation) and this may increase the likelihood of medication misadventure. Once again, however, the increased cost of maintaining a patient in a clinically stable state through regular outpatient or community-based contact with healthcare workers is still likely to be much cheaper than the cost of hospital admissions associated with recurrent clinical instability.[114]

The following is a broad overview of the pharmacological agents most commonly used in the management of chronic heart failure. It is important to note, however, that the nature of medical research, in respect to the diversity of scientific opinion and the constraints and vagaries of pharmaceutical company funding (resulting in selective examination of individual agents and recruitment of heterogeneous patient cohorts), means that many issues surrounding the optimal pharmacological management of chronic heart failure remain unresolved. In this context, Maseri et al. (1996)[118] have appropriately cautioned that individual needs often require rejection of the 'large-scale' evidence emanating from randomized controlled trials, simply because they fail to address an individual's particular circumstances.

Diuretics

Diuretic agents have long been the cornerstone of the pharmacological management of chronic heart failure. Loop diuretics (most commonly frusemide) are frequently used because of their ability to induce diuresis and therefore to reduce the symptoms of congestion by reducing preload.[79] Moreover, loop diuretics are less likely than thiazides to precipitate worsening renal dysfunction when co-prescribed with an ACE inhibitor.[119, 120] Overall, diuretics are commonly associated with symptomatic improvement and have been reported to reduce frequency of hospitalization.[121, 122] However, their effect on survival has never been examined in a randomized controlled study and, because of the ethical consideration of withdrawing what is now considered to be standard treatment, they are unlikely to be tested in this manner; especially as the clinical response to diuretic dosage tends to vary between patients. Patients frequently respond to the combination of frusemide and other types of diuretic including spironolactone, thiazides and metolazone.[123-5] For example, in severe heart failure, thiazides have been shown to have a synergistic effect with loop diuretics.[126] Most recently there has been increasing interest in the role of spironolactone in the management of chronic heart failure. Although spironolactone promotes less diuresis than frusemide it is an aldosterone antagonist and has a number of potential advantages when combined with a loop diuretic such as frusemide:

1. Enhanced diuresis.
2. Additional aldosterone inhibition above that of ACE inhibitors, which do not fully suppress aldosterone production in the typical setting of an activated renin-angiotensin-aldosterone system.[127, 128]
3. Growth factor inhibition.[62, 63]

On the basis of the potential value of spironolactone, a pilot study, the Randomised Aldactone Evaluation Study (RALES), examined the value of this agent among patients with chronic heart failure who had symptoms indicative of New York Heart Association (NYHA) Class III–IV, and found that active treatment with spironolactone was associated with an increase in both plasma renin activity and urinary aldosterone excretion and a decrease in atrial natriuretic factor.[64] A subsequent controlled study examining the effect of adjunctive spironolactone treatment on survival among patients with severe chronic heart failure was terminated prematurely as a result of significant mortality benefits associated with the study treatment, [129] and it has now become part of the standard pharmacological management of patients with severe chronic heart failure – although not without some controversy owing to higher adverse effects than first anticipated. This problem once again highlights the difficulty of extrapolating clinical trial results to the real patient population – especially when they are older, there is a more even gender balance and greater levels of comorbidity.[130]

Angiotensin-converting enzyme inhibitors

As discussed, patients with severe congestive heart failure in particular are likely to have increased renin-angiotensin-aldosterone system activity, resulting in greater concentrations of angiotensin II and aldosterone and therefore increased preload and afterload through greater vasoconstriction and sodium and water retention.[3] By decreasing the production of angiotensin II and inhibiting bradykinin catabolism, ACE inhibitors are thought to have a number of beneficial effects, including:

1. Decreased cardiac preload and afterload.
2. Prevention of ventricular remodelling.
3. Decreased catabolism of bradykinin
4. Improved endothelial function and reduced oxidative stress.[131]

In the context of severe congestive heart failure, the CONSENSUS trial was the first study to show that ACE inhibitors (in this case enalapril) have the potential to improve survival among such individuals, with about a 50% reduction in the risk of death at both 6 and 12 months associated with this agent in patients with severe heart failure.[132] More recent data, representing a 10-year follow-up of almost all the original cohort participating in the study, showed that the beneficial effects of enalapril in respect to survival were maintained for several years and the overall survival time was prolonged by about half.[133] These data do not reveal, however, whether the prolonged survival among treatment patients resulted in a comparable number of hospital admissions to that of control patients, although the authors assume that this did not occur. The results of this landmark study have been repeated in a number of subsequent studies that have consistently shown that ACE inhibitors improve survival and reduce hospital use among patients with moderate to severe chronic heart failure.[134, 135] Moreover, the results of the recent ATLAS study[136] suggest that a higher dose of lisinopril (up to 35 mg/day and therefore comparable to the level of ACE inhibition achieved in the previously mentioned clinical trials) was associated with a reduced incidence of death plus all-cause hospitalization as well as fewer admissions for heart failure in comparison with a low dose of lisinopril (2.5–5 mg/day and therefore more comparable to the level of ACE inhibition typically used in clinical practice).

Beta-adrenoceptor blockers

The most promising development in the management of heart failure in recent years (pending a prolonged critique of the impact of adjunctive spironolactone treatment in the management of severe heart failure[129]) has been the establishment of therapeutic benefit with various β-adrenoceptor blockers. These agents have long held the interest of clinicians for their ability to inhibit sympathetic nervous system activation and to theoretically combat the progression of heart failure. The first multicentre trials of β-adrenoceptor blockers in heart failure (the Metoprolol in Dilated Cardiomyopathy trial[137] and the Cardiac Insufficiency Bisoprolol I Study[138]) suggested that these agents improved left ventricular function and the clinical status of patients with heart failure. Moreover, they reduced the need for cardiac transplantation. More recently, studies in both the US[139] and Australia[140] showed that carvedilol (a β-adrenoceptor blocker with ancillary vasodilatory and antioxidant properties) was associated with reduced hospitalization, improved left ventricular function and probably survival among patients with mild to moderate heart failure. In this context, further studies, the Cardiac Insufficiency Bisoprolol Study (CIBIS-II)[141] and the Metoprolol CR/XL Randomised Intervention trial in Heart Failure (MERIT-HF)[142] have not only shown the ability of other beta blockers to reduce morbidity and mortality in patients with mild to moderate heart failure, but that such treatment is associated with lower healthcare costs.[143]

Most recently, the COPERNICUS Study has shown that adjunctive treatment of severe chronic heart failure with carvedilol was associated with improved survival and reduced morbidity. During an average of 10.4 months follow-up, adjunctive treatment with carvedilol was associated with a 35% survival benefit and a 24% decrease in the risk of death or hospitalization relative to the placebo arm of the study.[144] Because severe heart failure is usually associated with greater hospitalization rates, the relative cost-effectiveness of carvedilol treatment is likely to be greater than that associated with the adjunctive treatment of mild to moderate heart failure.

Digoxin

Digoxin has been used extensively in the management of chronic heart failure owing to the following beneficial effects:

1. Modulation of neurohormonal activity[145] resulting in decreased serum norepinephrine concentration[146, 147], improved baroreceptor function[147] and an overall decrease in sympathetic activity.[148]
2. Electrophysiological effects, resulting in a decrease in atrio-ventricular nodal conduction and control of the ventricular conduction rate in patients with atrial fibrillation.[149, 150]
3. Positive inotropic effects mediated through Na^+ K^+-ATPase inhibition.[151]

Despite its traditional use in chronic heart failure (although not without controversy), a definitive controlled study of the effects of digoxin among patients with mild to moderate chronic heart failure in sinus rhythm and receiving ACE inhibitors was only recently completed in 1997. The DIG Study demonstrated no effect on mortality.[152] However, digoxin was associated with reduced hospital use, especially that primarily associated with heart failure, and it seemed to have the most benefit in patients with more severe chronic heart failure. A number of studies[153, 154] have shown that digoxin seems to have the most benefit in patients with more severe heart failure, and that it is associated with poorer health outcomes if it is withdrawn suddenly. As such, digoxin differs from all of the other oral pharmacological agents with positive inotropic properties, such as amrinone, milrinone, enoximone and xamoterol, that have been proven in controlled studies to increase mortality when used to treat patients with chronic heart failure.[155]

Nitrates

Before the widespread introduction of the ACE inhibitors, the combination of hydralazine and nitrates was shown in the V-HeFT-II trial to marginally improve survival in patients with mild to moderate heart failure.[156] So, this combination represented the standard vasodilatory treatment for patients with chronic heart failure, prior to ACE inhibitors, and is recommended for use when ACE inhibition is contraindicated.[157] Considering that heart failure is commonly precipitated by ischaemic changes in the myocardium and that patients with chronic heart failure often need management of symptomatic ischaemic heart disease, concurrent nitrate therapy is common among patients with chronic heart failure. Although the effects of nitrates alone in chronic heart failure have not been examined in a controlled trial, there is some evidence to suggest that they do have some beneficial effects[158, 159], although the likelihood and subsequent consequence of 'nitrate tolerance' remains the same.[160, 161]

Calcium-channel antagonists

Many calcium-channel antagonists such as diltiazem[162] and nifedipine[163] have been shown to convey poorer health outcomes among patients with heart failure, most probably because of their negative inotropic effects.[78] More recently, however, the results of the PRAISE Study suggested that amlodipine was associated with no changes in mortality among patients with chronic heart failure while conveying possible benefit in the absence of myocardial ischaemia; [164] a follow-up study is currently examining this possible benefit prospectively.

Angiotensin II receptor (AT I) antagonists

Although the current pharmacotherapeutics used in the management of heart failure have been shown to generally improve health outcomes among patients with chronic heart failure, the overall limitations of their therapeutic effect, even in clinical trials, have resulted in a continual interest in the development and subsequent study of new therapeutic agents, of which there are many. Some of the most prominent and potentially effective of these are the angiotensin II receptor (AT I) antagonists. Interest in the therapeutic benefits of suppression of angiotensin II effect in heart failure arose from the observation that angiotensin II levels increase after prolonged treatment with ACE inhibitors, theoretically reducing their beneficial effects.[165] A number of studies examining angiotensin II receptor antagonists, with or without an ACE inhibitor, versus an ACE inhibitor alone are under way. Furthermore, the ELITE pilot study, [166] which compared treatment with losartan and captopril in the management of elderly patients with heart failure, gave some positive evidence in favour of losartan. For example, losartan was associated with a significant reduction in all-cause mortality (the primary end-point) and with a borderline reduction in the combined end-point of deaths and hospital admissions related to heart failure.

New studies likely to influence current practice

Although the ELITE pilot Study was favourable[166], the appropriately powered ELITE-II Study showed no incremental benefits of losartan over treatment with captopril.[167] At the time of this book, therefore, it is assumed that AII inhibitors are indicated only if ACE inhibitors are contraindicated, although this needs to be confirmed formally – this represents one of the arms of the CHARM Study, which includes arms that are comparing candersartan (an AII inhibitor) versus placebo in patients intolerant to ACE inhibition with and without left ventricular systolic dysfunction and combined ACE and AII inhibition versus ACE alone. Alternatively, the HEAAL Study will compare high versus low levels of losartan versus ACE alone. In this context, the Val-Heft Study (reported at the 'hot-line' session of the AHA meeting in New Orleans in November 2000) showed that combined valsartan (an AII inhibitor) and ACE inhibition was more beneficial than ACE inhibition alone. However, a sub-analysis of the data suggested that patients receiving a beta blocker fared worse – therefore, these data are unlikely to be applied on a clinical basis until the CHARM Study has been completed (which is most likely to be reported at either the AHA meeting in late 2001 or the ACC meeting in early 2002). At around the same time, it is likely that the OVERTURE Study (comparing omapatrilat, a dual action, vasopeptidase inhibitor) will be reported and will indicate whether such adjunctive therapy should be added to the current gold standard treatment of heart failure. Two recently aborted trials (RENAISSANCE AND RECOVER) have provided strong evidence that treatment with anti-cytokines is unlikely to provide another avenue of treatment for heart failure.[168] Alternatively, the fate of endothelin-1 receptor antagonists remains unknown after the positive REACH-1[169] but negative ENCOR studies.

Pharmacological overview

Clearly, the pharmacological management of heart failure is an evolving field, albeit one driven by commercial rather than altruistic concerns in many cases. New treatments are likely to target ancillary issues in the management of heart failure (for example, the WASH Study, which is examining the benefits of antico-agulation/anti-platelet treatment[170]). Bi-ventricular pacing, in order to provide better synchronization of the cardiac cycle in the setting of underlying heart failure, has been shown in preliminary studies (for example, the MIRACLE Study[167]) to provide clinical benefits and is the subject of appropriately powered, large-scale randomized studies (for example, the CARE-HF and COMPANION studies).[167] Although it difficult to even predict the gold-standard treatment of heart failure in the year 2005 (that is, in a time frame in which evidence from these trials will be incorporated into management guidelines), it is quite clear that the overall management of heart failure will become increasingly complicated, with many therapeutic options available to the clinician.

Current deficiencies in the management of severe congestive heart failure

Although the outlook may be brighter, there is ample evidence to suggest that the current armoury of pharmacological agents used in the longer-term management of severe congestive heart failure have failed to fully ameliorate the morbidity and mortality associated with this debilitating syndrome. For example, in the Studies of Left Ventricular Dysfunction (SOLVD) treatment trial, 35% of patients in the enalapril group died within 3.5 years of follow-up, 46% were admitted to hospital with worsening chronic heart failure and 69% were admitted to hospital for any reason.[171, 172]

As such, chronic heart failure remains a common cause of disability (with associated poorer levels of health-related quality of life) and death.[173–9] It is also characterized, in a proportion of severe cases, by extensive hospital use[173–9], which, as discussed, is a considerable burden on the healthcare system, accounting for about two-thirds of the overall costs needed to manage such patients and 1–2% of overall healthcare expenditure.[109, 110] The relative inadequacy of the current management of heart failure overall is best illustrated by the recent data from studies examining the pattern of hospital use among relatively unselected (and therefore predominantly older) cohorts of patients admitted to hospital with congestive heart failure. In these studies, the reported all-cause readmission rates range from 25% to 47%[177–83] within three months of discharge, and 33% to 54%[175–7, 184] within six months of discharge from acute hospitalization.

Summary

Heart failure is a growing health problem. Currently available pharmacological treatment strategies do not completely ameliorate the high morbidity and mortality associated with chronic heart failure, especially in older people. There is a clear need, therefore, to develop and implement cost-effective programmes that prevent the development of heart failure (for example, primary prevention in coronary heart disease). There is also a need for programmes that provide for the early detection and treatment of individuals who develop heart failure despite prevention strategies (for example, screening with echocardiography or elevated naturietic peptide levels).

Unfortunately, the most urgent need relates to the increasing number of older individuals with chronic heart failure who are being hospitalized. There is strong evidence to suggest that such individuals have limited survival prospects and are likely to have extremely poor quality of life and to require recurrent hospitalization before they die. Chapter 3 describes epidemiological studies examining the modern-day burden of heart failure in the whole Scottish population – a typical developed country.

It is in this overall context that specialist-nurse intervention programmes have the potential to limit the overall burden of chronic heart failure by limiting costly hospital admissions, in addition to improving quality of life on an individual basis by providing more tailored and attentive health care. Studies examining the potential benefits of these programmes are described in Chapters 4 and 5.

References

1.   Kelly D. Our future society: A global challenge. *Circulation* 1997; 95: 2459–64.
2.   Denolin H, Kuhn H, Krayenbuehl H, et al. The definition of heart failure. *Eur Heart J* 1983; 4: 445–8.
3.   Packer M. Pathophysiology of chronic heart failure. *Lancet* 1992; 340: 88–95.
4.   Hoes A, Mosterd A, Grobbee DE. An epidemic of heart failure? Recent evidence from Europe. *Eur Heart J* 1998; 19: L2–L8.
5.   Atherton J, Thomson H, Moore T, et al. Diastolic ventricular interaction: A possible mechanism for abnormal vascular responses during volume unloading in heart failure. *Circulation* 1997; 96: 4273–9.
6.   Atherton J, Moore T, Thomson H, et al. Restrictive left ventricular filling patterns are predictive of diastolic ventricular interaction in chronic heart failure. *J Am Coll Cardiol* 1998; 1: 413–18.
7.   The World Health Organization/Council on Geriatric Cardiology Task Force on Heart Failure Education. Concise guide to the management of heart failure. *Am J Geriatr Cardiol* 1996; 5: 13–30.
8.   Cowie M, Wood DA, Coats AJ, et al. Incidence and aetiology of heart failure: A population based study. *Eur Heart J* 1999; 20: 421–8.
9.   Baig K, Niall M, McKenna W, et al. The pathophysiology of advanced heart failure. *Am Heart J* 1998; 135 (suppl): S216–S30.
10.   Cowburn P, Cleland J, Coats A, et al. Risk stratification in chronic heart failure. *Eur Heart J* 1998; 19: 696–710.
11.   Dougherty A, Naccarelli G, Gray E, et al. Congestive heart failure with normal systolic function. *Am J Cardiol* 1984; 54: 778–82.
12.   Braunwald E. Pathophysiology of heart failure. In: Braunwald E, ed. *Heart Disease.* 4th ed. Philadelphia, PA: W.B. Saunders, 1992: 393–418.
13.   Mulieri L, Hasenfuss G, Leavitt B, et al. Altered myocardial force-frequency relation in human heart failure. *Circulation* 1992; 85: 1743–50.
14.   Hasenfuss G, Holubarsch C, Hermann H, et al. Influence of the force-frequency relationship on haemodynamics and left ventricular function in patients with non-failing hearts and in patients with dilated cardiomyopathy. *Eur Heart J* 1994; 15: 164–70.

15. Connelly C, McLaughlin R, Vogel W, et al. Reversible and irreversible elongation of ischemic, infarcted and healed myocardium in response to increases in preload and afterload. *Circulation* 1991; 84: 387–99.

16. Sharpe N. Ventricular remodelling following myocardial infarction. *Am J Cardiol* 1992; 70 (suppl): 20C–26C.

17. Nadal-Ginard B, Mahdavi V. Molecular basis of cardiac performance: Plasticity of the myocardium generated through protein isoform switches. *J Clin Invest* 1989; 84: 1693–700.

18. Messerli F. *Pathophysiology of Left Ventricular Hypertrophy*. London: Science Press, 1992.

19. Anversa P, Ricci R, Olivetti G. Quantitative structural analysis of the myocardium during physiologic growth and induced cardiac hypertrophy: A review. *J Am Coll Cardiol* 1986; 7: 1140–9.

20. Weber K, Sun Y, Campbell S. Structural remodelling of the heart by fibrous tissue: Role of circulating hormones and locally produced peptides. *Eur Heart J* 1995; 16 (suppl): N12–N18.

21. Beltrami C, Finato N, Rocco M, et al. Structural basis of end-stage failure in ischemic cardiomyopathy in humans. *Circulation* 1995; 89: 151–63.

22. Geisterfer A, Peach M, Owens G. Angiotensin II induces hypertrophy, not hyperplasia, of cultured rat aortic smooth muscle cells. *Circ Res* 1988; 62: 749–56.

23. Geisterfer A, Owens G. Arginine vasopressin-induced hypertrophy of cultured rat aortic smooth muscle cells. *Hypertension* 1989; 14: 413–20.

24. Simpson P, McGrath A. Norepinephrine-stimulated hypertrophy of cultured rat myocardial cells in alpha 1-adrenergic response. *J Clin Invest* 1983; 72: 732–8.

25. Olivetti G, Abbi R, Quaini F, et al. Apoptosis in the failing human heart. *New Engl J Med* 1997; 336: 1131–41.

26. Testa M, Yeh M, Lee P, et al. Circulating levels of cytokines and their endogenous modulators in patients with mild to severe congestive heart failure due to coronary artery disease or hypertension. *Circulation* 1996; 28: 964–71.

27. Morgan H, Baker K. Cardiac hypertrophy: Mechanical, neural and endocrine dependence. *Circulation* 1991; 83: 13–18.

28. Creager M, Faxon D, Cutler S, et al. Contribution of vasopressin to vasoconstriction in patients with congestive heart failure: Comparison with renin-angiotensin system and the sympathetic nervous system. *J Am Coll Cardiol* 1986; 7: 758–65.

29. Margulies K, Hilderbrand F, Lerman A, et al. Increased endothelin in experienced heart failure. *Circulation* 1990; 82: 2226–30.

30. Kubo S, Rector T, Bank A, et al. Endothelium-dependent vasodilation is attenuated in patients with heart failure. *Circulation* 1991; 84: 1589–96.

31. Cody R, Atlas S, Laragh L, et al. Atrial natiuretic factor in normal subjects and heart failure patients: Plasma levels and renal, hormonal, and hemodynamic responses to peptide infusion. *J Clin Invest* 1986; 78: 1362–74.

32. Hirooka Y, Takeshita A, Imaizumi T, et al. Attenuated forearm vasodilative response to intra-arterial atrial natiuretic peptide in heart failure. *Circulation* 1990; 82: 147–53.

33. Dzau V. Vascular and renal prostaglandins as counter-regulatory systems in heart failure. *Eur Heart J* 1988; 9 (suppl): H15–H19.

34. Heerdink E, Leufkens H, Herings R, et al. NSAIDs associated with increased risk of congestive heart failure in elderly patients taking diuretics. *Arch Intern Med* 1998; 158: 1108–12.

35.   Leri A, Liu Y, Malhotra A. Pacing-induced heart failure in dogs enhances the expression of p53 and p53-dependent genes in ventricular myocytes. *Circulation* 1998; 97: 194–203.

36.   Torre-Amione G, Kapadia S, Lee J, et al. Tumor necrosis factor-alpha and tumor necrosis factor in severe chronic heart failure. *Circulation* 1996; 93: 704–11.

37.   Torre-Amione G, Kapadia S, Lee J, et al. Expression and functional significance of tumor necrosis factor receptors in human myocardium. *Circulation* 1995; 92: 1487–93.

38.   McDonagh T, Morrison C, Lawrence C, et al. Symptomatic and asymptomatic left-ventricular systolic dysfunction in an urban population. *Lancet* 1997; 350: 829–33.

39.   Adams K, Zannard F. Clinical definition and epidemiology of advanced heart failure. *Am Heart J* 1998; 135: S204–15.

40.   Colucci W, Braunwald E. Pathophysiology of heart failure. In: Braunwald E, ed. *Heart Disease.* 5th ed. Philadelphia, PA: W.B. Saunders, 1997: 394–420.

41.   Chakko C, Woska D, Martinez H, et al. Clinical, radiographic, and hemodynamic correlations in chronic congestive heart failure. *Am J Med* 1991; 90: 353–9.

42.   Stevenson L, Perloff J. The limited reliability of physical signs for the estimation of hemodynamics in chronic heart failure. *JAMA* 1989; 261: 884–8.

43.   Stevenson L, Massie B, Francis G. Optimizing therapy for complex or refractory heart failure: A management algorithm. *Am Heart J* 1998; 135: S293–309.

44.   Borow K, Neumann A, Wynne J. Sensitivity of end-systolic pressure-dimension and pressure-volume relations to the inotropic state in humans. *Circulation* 1982; 65: 988–97.

45.   Lamas G, Vaughan D, Parisi A, et al. Effects of left ventricular shape and captopril therapy on exercise capacity after anterior wall acute myocardial infarction. *Am J Cardiol* 1989; 63: 1167–73.

46.   Cohn JN, Johnson G, Ziesche S. A comparison of enalapril with hydralazine-isosorbide dinitrate in the treatment of chronic congestive heart failure. *N Engl J Med* 1991; 325: 293–302.

47.   The CONSENSUS Trial Study Group. Effects of enalapril on mortality in severe congestive heart failure: Results of the Cooperative North Scandinavian Enalapril Survival Study (CONSENSUS). *N Engl J Med* 1987; 316: 1429–35.

48.   Stevenson W, Stevenson L, Middlekauff H, et al. Sudden death prevention in patients with advanced ventricular dysfunction. *Circulation* 1993; 88: 2953–61.

49.   Wilt A, Janse M. Experimental models of ventricular tachycardia and fibrillation caused by ischemia and infarction. *Circulation* 1992; 85: 132–42.

50.   Cohn J, Levine T, Olivari M, et al. Plasma norepinephrine as a guide to prognosis in patients with chronic congestive heart failure. *N Engl J Med* 1984; 311: 819–23.

51.   Packer M, Lee W. Provocation of hyper and hypokalemia sudden death during treatment with and withdrawal of converting-enzyme inhibition in severe chronic congestive heart failure. *Am J Cardiol* 1986; 57: 347–8.

52.   Archie J. Transmural distribution of intrinsic and transmitted left ventricular diastolic intramyocardial pressure in dogs. *Cardiovasc Res* 1978; 12: 255–62.

53.   Bache R, Cobb F. Effect of maximal coronary vasodilation on transmural myocardial perfusion during tachycardia in the awake dog. *Circ Res* 1977; 41: 648–53.

54.   Bellamy R, Lowensohn H, Olsson R. Factors determining delayed peak flow in canine myocardial reactive hyperaemia. *Cardiovasc Res* 1979; 13: 147–150.

55.   Unverferth D, Magorien R, Lewis R, et al. The role of subendocardial ischemia in perpetuating myocardial failure in patients with non-ischemic congestive cardiomyopathy. *Am Heart J* 1983; 105: 176–9.

56. Ferrari R, Agnoletti L, Comini L, et al. Oxidative stress during myocardial ischaemia and heart failure. *Eur Heart J* 1998; 19 (suppl): B2–B11.

57. Ferrari R, Bongrazio M, Cargnoni A, et al. Heat shock protein changes in hibernation: A similarity with heart failure. *J Mol Cell Cardiol* 1996; 28: 2383–95.

58. Blitz A, Laks H. The role of coronary revascularization in the management of heart failure: Identification of candidates and review of results. *Curr Opin Cardiol* 1996; 11: 276–90.

59. Beltrami C, Finato N, Rocco M, et al. The cellular basis of dilated cardiomyopathy in humans. *J Mol Cell Cardiol* 1995; 27: 291–305.

60. Kajstura J, Zhang X, Liu Y, et al. The cellular basis of pacing-induced dilated cardiomy-opathy. Myocyte cell loss and myocyte cellular reactive hypertrophy. *Circulation* 1995; 92: 2306–17.

61. Tan L, Jalil J, Pick R, et al. Cardiac myocyte necrosis induced by angiotensin II. *Circ Res* 1991; 69: 1185–95.

62. Young M, Fullerton M, Dilley R, Funder J. Mineralocorticoids, hypertension and cardiac fibrosis. *J Clin Invest* 1994; 93: 2578.

63. Hall C, Hall O. Hypertension and hypersalimentation. I. Aldosterone hypertension. *Lab Invest* 1965; 14: 285.

64. The RALES Investigators. Effectiveness of spirinolactone added to an angiotensin-con-verting enzyme inhibitor and a loop-diuretic for severe chronic congestive heart failure. *Am J Cardiol* 1996; 78: 902–7.

65. Harris P. Congestive cardiac failure: Central role of the arterial blood pressure. *Br Heart J* 1987; 58: 190–203.

66. Vanhoutte P. Adjustments in the peripheral circulation in chronic heart failure. *Eur Heart J* 1983; 4 (suppl): A67–A70.

67. Drexler H, Hayoz D, Munzel T, et al. Endothelial function in congestive heart failure. *Am Heart J* 1993; 126: 761–4.

68. Kaiser L, Spickard R, Olivier N. Heart failure depresses endothelium-dependent responses in canine femoral artery. *Am J Physiol* 1989; 256 (suppl): H962–H67.

69. Wei C, Lerman A, Rodeheffer R, et al. Endothelin in human congestive heart failure. *Circulation* 1994; 89: 1580–6.

70. Szlachcic J, Massie B, Kramer B. Correlates and prognostic implication of exercise capacity in chronic congestive heart failure. *Am J Cardiol* 1985; 55: 1037–42.

71. Franciosa J, Park M, Levine T. Lack of correlation between exercise capacity and indexes of resting left ventricular performance in heart failure. *Am J Cardiol* 1981; 47: 33–9.

72. Anker S, Coats A. Syndrome of cardiac cachexia. In: Poole-Wilson P, Colucci W, Massie B, et al., eds. *Heart Failure*. New York: Churchill Livingstone, 1997: 261–7.

73. Anker S, Coats A. Cachexia in heart failure is bad for you. *Eur Heart J* 1998; 19: 191–3.

74. Otaki M. Surgical treatment of patients with cardiac cachexia. An analysis of factors affecting operative mortality. *Chest* 1994; 105: 1347–51.

75. Anker S, Ponikowski P, Varney S, et al. Wasting as independent risk factor of survival in chronic heart failure. *Lancet* 1997; 349: 1050–3.

76. Fonarow G, Chelimsky-Fallick C, Stevenson L, et al. Effect of direct vasodilatation with hydralazine versus angiotensin-converting enzyme inhibition with captopril on mortality in advanced heart failure. *J Am Coll Cardiol* 1992; 19: 842–50.

77. Steimle A, Stevenson L, Chelimsky-Fallick C, et al. Sustained hemodynamic efficacy of therapy tailored to reduce filling pressures in survivors with advanced heart failure. *Circulation* 1997; 96: 1165–72.

78. Gheorhiade M, Cody R, Francis G, et al. Current medical therapy for advanced heart failure. *Am Heart J* 1998; 135 (suppl): S231–48.

79. O'Connor C, Gattis W, Swedburg K. Current and novel pharmacological approaches in advanced heart failure. *Am Heart J* 1998; 135 (suppl): S249–263.

80. Bonneux L, Barendregt J, Meeter K, et al. Estimating clinical morbidity due to ischemic heart disease and congestive heart failure: The future rise of heart failure. *Am J Public Health* 1994; 84: 20–8.

81. Schocken D, Arrieta M, Leaverton P, et al. Prevalence and mortality rate of congestive heart failure in the United States. *J Am Coll Cardiol* 1992; 20: 301–6.

82. Mair F, Crowley T, Bundred P. Prevalence, aetiology and management of heart failure in general practice. *Br J Gen Pract* 1996; 46: 77–9.

83. Gillum R. Epidemiology of heart failure in the United States. *Am Heart J* 1993; 126: 1042–6.

84. Ghali J, Cooper R, Ford E. Trends in hospitalization rates for heart failure in the United States, 1973–1986. *Arch Intern Med* 1990; 150: 769–73.

85. Ho K, Anderson K, Kannel W, et al. Survival after the onset of congestive heart failure in Framingham Heart Study subjects. *Circulation* 1993; 88: 107–15.

86. Ho KK, Pinsky JL, Kannel WB, et al. The epidemiology of heart failure: The Framingham Study. *J Am Coll Cardiol* 1993; 22 (4 Suppl A): 6A–13A.

87. Eriksson H, Svardsudd K, Larsson B, et al. Risk factors for heart failure in the general population: The study of men born in 1913. *Eur Heart J* 1989; 10: 647–56.

88. Remes J, Reunanen A, Aromaa A, et al. Incidence of heart failure in eastern Finland: A population-based surveillance study. *Eur Heart J* 1992; 13: 588–93.

89. Royal College of General Practitioners and Department of Health and Social Security. *Morbidity Statistics from General Practice: Fourth National Study, 1991–92*. London: HSMO, 1995.

90. Van de Lisdonk E, Van den Bosch WJ, Huygen F, et al. *Diseases in General Practice*. Bunge: Utrecht, 1990.

91. Lamberts H, Brouwer H, Mohrs J. *Reason for Encounter – And Episode and Process -oriented Standard Output from the Transition Project. Part 1 & 2*. Amsterdam: Department of General Practice, 1993.

92. Rodeheffer R, Jacobsen S, Gersh B, et al. The incidence and prevalence of congestive heart failure in Rochester. *Mayo Clin Proc* 1993; 68: 1143–50.

93. Gibson T, White K, Klainer L. The prevalence of congestive heart failure in two rural communities. *J Chronic Dis* 1966; 19: 141–52.

94. Cowie M, Mosterd A, Wood DA, et al. The epidemiology of heart failure. *Eur Heart J* 1997; 18: 208–25.

95. Klainer L, Gibson T, White K. The epidemiology of cardiac failure. *J Chronic Dis* 1966; 19: 141–52.

96. Erikson H, Wilhelmsen B, Herlitz J. Epidemiology and prognosis of heart failure. *Z Kardiol* 1991; 80 (Suppl 8): 831–6.

97. Dinkel R, Buchner K, Holtz J. Chronic heart failure. Socioeconomic relevance in the Federal Republic of Germany. *Munch Med Wschr* 1989; 131: 686–89.

98. Koopmanschap M, van Roijen L, Bonneux L. *Costs of Diseases in the Netherlands*. Report of the Department of Public Health and Social Medicine and the Institute for Medical Technology Assessment. Rotterdam: Erasmus University, 1992.

99. McMurray J, McDonagh T, Morrison CE, et al. Trends in hospitalization for heart failure in Scotland 1980–1990. *Eur Heart J* 1993; 14: 1158–62.

100. Rodriguez-Artalejo F, Guallar-Castillon P, Banegas B, et al. Trends in hospitalization and mortality for heart failure in Spain, 1980–1993. *Eur Heart J* 1997; 18: 1771–9.

101. Ranofsky A. *Inpatient Utilization of Short-stay Hospitals by Diagnosis.* National Center for Health Statistics, Vital and Health Statistics. Washington, DC: US Department of Health, Education, and Welfare, 1974.

102. Graves E. *Detailed Diagnoses and Procedures, National Hospital Discharge Survey, 1990.* National Center for Health Statistics, Vital and Health Statistics. Washington, DC: US Department of Health and Human Services, 1991.

103. Lenfant C. Report of the Task Force on Research in Heart Failure. *Circulation* 1994; 90: 1118–23.

104. Croft JB, Giles WH, Pollard RA, et al. National trends in the initial hospitalization for heart failure. *J Am Geriatr Soc* 1997; 45: 270–5.

105. Kannel W, Ho K, Thom T. Changing epidemiological features of cardiac failure. *Br Heart J* 1994; 72 (suppl): S3–S9.

106. Garg R, Packer M, Pitt B, et al. Heart failure in the 1990s: Evolution of a major public health problem in cardiovascular medicine. *J Am Coll Cardiol* 1993(suppl A); 22: 3A–5A.

107. Graves EJ. *1989 Summary: National Hospital Discharge Survey. Advance Data from Vital and Health Statistics. No. 199.* Hyattsville, MD: Public Health Service, 1991.

108. Yamani M, Massie B. Congestive heart failure: Insights from epidemiology, implications. *Mayo Clin Proc* 1993; 68: 214–18.

109. McMurray J, Hart W, Rhodes G. An evaluation of the cost of heart failure to the National Health Service in the UK. *Br J Med Econ* 1993; 6: 99–110.

110. McMurray JJV, Stewart S. Epidemiology, aetiology and prognosis of heart failure. *Heart* 2000; 83: 596–602.

111. van Hout B, Wielink G, Bonsel G, et al. Effects of ACE inhibitors in the Netherlands: A pharmaco-economic model. *PharmacoEconomics* 1993; 3: 387–97.

112. Launois R, Launois B, Reboul-Marty J, et al. Le coût de la sévérité de la malaidie: Le cas de l'insuffisance-cardiaque. *J Econ Med* 1990; 8: 395–412.

113. O'Connell J, Bristow M. Economic impact of heart failure in the United States: Time for a different approach. *J Heart Lung Transplant* 1993; 13: S107–S12.

114. Mark DB. Economics of treating heart failure. *Am J Cardiol* 1997; 80(8B): 33H–38H.

115. Rich MW. Epidemiology, pathophysiology, and etiology of congestive heart failure in older adults. *J Am Geriatr Soc* 1997; 45: 968–74.

116. Oka R. Physiological changes in heart failure – 'What's new'. *J Cardiovasc Nurs* 1996; 10: 11–28.

117. Hart W, Rhodes G, McMurray J. The cost effectiveness of enalapril in the treatment of chronic heart failure. *Br J Med Econ* 1993; 6: 91–8.

118. Maseri A, Cianflone D, Pasceri V, et al. The risk and cost-effectiveness of individual patient management: The challenge of a new generation of clinical trials. *Cardiovasc Drugs Ther* 1996; 10: 751–8.

119. Baker D, Constam M, Bottoft M, et al. Management of heart failure. Pharmacological treatment. *JAMA* 1994; 272: 1361–6.

120. Williams J, Bristow M, Fowler M, et al. Guidelines for the evaluation and management of heart failure. Report of the American College of Cardiology/American Heart Association Task Force on Practice Guidelines (Committee on Evaluation and Management of Heart Failure). *J Am Coll Cardiol* 1995; 26: 1376–98.

121. Richardson A, Bayliss J, Scriven A, et al. Double blind comparison of captopril alone against furosemide plus amiloride in mild heart failure. *Lancet* 1987; 2: 709–11.

122. Dyckner T, Wester P. Salt and water balance in congestive heart failure. *Acta Med Scand* 1986; 707 (suppl): 27–31.

123. Cleland J, Gillen G, Dargie J. The effects of frusemide and angiotensin-converting enzyme inhibitors and the combination on cardiac and renal hemodynamics in heart failure. *Eur Heart J* 1988; 9: 132–41.

124. Dahlstrom U, Karlsson E. Captopril and spirinolactone therapy for refractory congestive heart failure. *Am J Cardiol* 1993; 71 (suppl): 29A–33A.

125. Vasko M, Cartwright D, Knochel J, et al. Furosemide absorption altered in decompensated congestive heart failure. *Ann Intern Med* 1985; 102: 314–18.

126. Channer K, McLean K, Lawson-Matthew P, et al. Combination diuretic treatment in severe heart failure: A randomised controlled trial. *Br Heart J* 1994; 71: 146–50.

127. Marayev V, Skvortsov A, Masenko V, et al. Escape of ACE inhibitor effects on aldosterone during long-term treatment of congestive heart failure. *International Meeting on Heart Failure.* Amsterdam: April, 1995.

128. Straessen J, Lijnen P, Fagard R, et al. Rise in plasma concentration of aldosterone during long-term angiotensin II suppression. *J Endocrinol* 1981; 91: 457–65.

129. Pitt B, Zannad F, Remme WJ, et al. The effect of spironolactone on morbidity and mortality in patients with severe heart failure. Randomized Aldactone Evaluation Study Investigators. *N Engl J Med* 1999; 341: 709–17.

130. Petrie M, Berry C, Stewart S, et al. Older hearts in failure. *Eur Heart J* (in press).

131. Tewksbury D. Angiotensinogen: Biochemistry and molecular biology. In: Laragh J, Brenner B, eds. *Hypertension: Pathophysiology, Diagnosis and Management.* New York: Raven Press, 1990: 1197–216.

132. The CONSENSUS Trial Study Group. Effects of enalapril on mortality in severe congestive heart failure: Results of the Cooperative North Scandinavian Enalapril Survival Study (CONSENSUS). *N Engl J Med* 1987; 316: 1429–35.

133. Swedberg K, Kjekshus J, Snapinn S, for the CONSENSUS Investigators. Long-term survival in severe heart failure in patients with enalapril. *Eur Heart J* 1999; 20: 136–9.

134. The SOLVD Investigators. Effect of enalapril on survival in patients with reduced left ventricular ejection fractions and congestive heart failure. *N Engl J Med* 1991; 325: 293–302.

135. Chalmers J, West M, Cryan J, et al. Placebo-controlled study of lisinopril in congestive heart failure: A multicentre study. *J Cardiovasc Pharmacol* 1987; 9 (suppl): S89–S97.

136. Packer M, Poole-Wilson PA, Armstrong PW, et al. Comparative effects of low and high doses of the angiotensin converting enzyme inhibitor, lisinopril, on morbidity and mortality in chronic heart failure. *Circulation* 1999; 100: 2312–18.

137. Waagstein F, Bristow M, Swedberg K, et al. Beneficial effects of metoprolol in idiopathic dilated cardiomyopathy. *Lancet* 1993; 342: 1441–6.

138. The CIBIS Investigators. A randomized trial of beta-blockade in heart failure: The Cardiac Insufficiency Bisoprolol Study (CIBIS). *Circulation* 1994; 90: 1765–73.

139. Packer M, Bristow M, Cohn J, for the US Carvedilol Group. The effect of carvedilol on morbidity and mortality in patients with chronic heart failure. *N Engl J Med* 1996; 334: 1349–55.

140. The Australia–New Zealand Heart Failure Research Collaborative Group. Effects of carvedilol, a vasodilator beta-blocker, in patients with congestive heart failure due to ischemic heart disease. *Circulation* 1995; 92: 212–18.

141. CIBIS II Investigators. The Cardiac Insufficiency Bisoprolol Study II (CIBIS II): A randomised trial. *Lancet* 1999; 353: 9–13.

142. Merit-HF Study Group. Effect of metoprolol CR/XL in chronic heart failure: Metoprolol CR/XL Randomized Intervention Trial in Congestive Heart Failure (MERIT-HF). *JAMA* 2000; 383: 1295–302.

143. CIBIS-II Investigators and Health Economics Group. Reduced costs with bisoprolol treatment for heart failure: An economic analysis of the second cardiac insufficiency bisoprolol study (CIBIS-II). *Eur Heart J*, in press.

144. Packer M, Coats AJS, Fowler MB, et al., for the Carvedilol Prospective Randomized Cumulative Survival (COPERNICUS) Study Group. Effect of carvedilol on survival in severe chronic heart failure. *N Engl J Med* 2001; 344: 1651–8.

145. Gheorghiade M, Ferguson D. Digoxin: A neurohormonal modulator in heart failure? *Circulation* 1991; 84: 2181–6.

146. Van Veldhuisen D, Man in't Veld A, Dunselman P, et al. Double-blind placebo-controlled study of ibopamine and digoxin in patients with mild to moderate heart failure: Results of the Dutch Ibopamine Multicentre Trial (DIMT). *J Am Coll Cardiol* 1993; 22: 1564–73.

147. Krum H, Bigger J, Goldsmith R, et al. Effect of long-term digoxin therapy on autonomic function in patients with chronic heart failure. *J Am Coll Cardiol* 1995; 25: 289–94.

148. Ferguson D, Berg W, Sanders J, et al. Sympathoinhibitory responses to digitalis glycosides in heart failure patients: Direct evidence from sympathetic neural recordings. *Circulation* 1989; 80: 65–77.

149. Redfors A. The effect of different doses on subjective symptoms and physical working capacity in patients with atrial fibrillation. *Act Med Scand* 1971; 190: 307–20.

150. Gold H, Cattel M, Greiner T, et al. Clinical pharmacology of digoxin. *J Pharmacol Exp Ther* 1953; 109: 45–57.

151. Powell A, Horowitz J, Hasin Y, et al. Acute myocardial uptake of digoxin in humans: Correlations with hemodynamic and electrocardiographic effects. *J Am Coll Cardiol* 1990; 15: 1238–47.

152. The Digitalis Investigation Group. The effect of digoxin on mortality and morbidity in patients with heart failure. *N Engl J Med* 1997; 336: 525–33.

153. Uretsky B, Young J, Shahidi F, et al. Randomized study assessing the effect of digoxin withdrawal in patients with mild to moderate chronic congestive heart failure: Results of the PROVED trial. *J Am Coll Cardiol* 1993; 22: 955–62.

154. Packer M, Gheorghiade M, Young J, et al. Withdrawal of digoxin from patients with chronic heart failure treated with angiotensisn-converting-enzyme inhibitors. *N Engl J Med* 1993; 329: 1–7.

155. Reddy S, Benatar D, Gheorghiade M. Update on digoxin and other oral positive inotropic agents for chronic heart failure. *Curr Opin Cardiol* 1997; 12: 233–41.

156. Cohn J, Archibald D, Ziesche S, et al. Effect of vasodilator therapy on mortality in chronic congestive heart failure: Results of a Veterans Administration Cooperative Study. *N Engl J Med* 1986; 314: 1547–52.

157. The ACC/AHA Task Force on Practice Guidelines (Committee on Evaluation and Management of Heart Failure). Guidelines for the evaluation and management of heart failure. *J Am Coll Cardiol* 1995; 26: 1376–98.

158. Leier C, Huss P, Magorien R, et al. Improved exercise capacity and differing arterial venous intolerance during chronic isosorbide dinitrate therapy for congestive heart failure. *Circulation* 1983; 67: 817–22.

159. Cohn J. Nitrates are effective in the treatment of chronic congestive heart failure: The protagonist's view. *Am J Cardiol* 1990; 66: 444–6.

160. Elkayam U, Roth A, Henriquez B, et al. The hemodynamic and hormonal effects of high dose transdermal nitroglycerin in patients with chronic congestive heart failure. *Am J Cardiol* 1985; 56: 555–9.

161. Elkayam U. Nitrates in the treatment of congestive heart failure. *Am J Cardiol* 1996; 77 (suppl): 41C–51C.

162. The Multicenter Diltiazem Postinfarction Trial Research Group. The effect of diltiazem on mortality and reinfarction after myocardial infarction. *N Engl J Med* 1988; 319: 385–93.

163. Elkayam U, Amin J, Mehra A, et al. A prospective, randomized, double-blind, crossover study to compare the efficacy and safety of chronic nifedipine therapy with that of isosorbide dinitrate and their combination in the treatment of chronic congestive heart failure. *Circulation* 1990; 82: 1954–61.

164. Packer M, O'Connor C, Ghali J, et al. Effect of Amlodipine on morbidity and mortality in severe chronic heart failure. *N Engl J Med* 1996; 335: 1107–14.

165. Pitt B, Chang P, Timmermans P. Angiotensin II receptor antagonists in heart failure: Rationale and design of the Evaluation of Losartan in the Elderly (ELITE) trial. *Cardiovasc Drug Ther* 1995; 9: 693–700.

166. Pitt B, Martinez F, Georg M, et al. Randomised trial of losartan versus captopril in patients over 65 with heart failure (Evaluation of Losartan in the Elderly Study, ELITE). *Lancet* 1997; 349: 747–52.

167. Pitt B, Poole-Wilson PA, Segal R, et al., on behalf of the ELITE-II Investigators. Effect of losartan compared with captopril on mortality in patients with symptomatic heart failure: Randomised trial – the Losartan Heart Failure Survival Study Elite-II. *Lancet* 2000; 355: 1582–7.

168. Louis A, Cleland JGF, Crabbe S, et al. Clinical trials update: CAPRICORN, COPERNICUS, MIRACLE, STAF, RITZ-2, RECOVER and RENAISSANCE and cachexia and cholesterol in heart failure. Highlights of the scientific sessions of the American College of Cardiology, 2001. *Eur J Heart Failure* 2001; 3: 381–7.

169. Mylona P, Cleland JGF. Update of REACH-1 and MERIT-HF clinical trials in heart failure. *Eur J Heart Failure* 1999; 1: 197–200.

170. Jones CG, Cleland JGF. Meeting report – The LIDO, HOPE, MOXCON, and WASH studies. *Eur J of Heart Failure* 1999; 1: 425–31.

171. The SOLVD Investigators. Effect of enalapril on survival in patients with reduced left ventricular ejection fractions and congestive heart failure. *N Engl J Med* 1991; 325: 293–302.

172. The SOLVD Investigators. Effect of enalapril on mortality and the development of heart failure in asymptomatic patients with reduced left ventricular ejection fractions. *N Engl J Med* 1992; 327: 685–91.

173. Gorkin L, Norvell NK, Rosen RC, et al. Assessment of quality of life as observed from the baseline data of the studies of left ventricular dysfunction (SOLVD) trial quality-of-life substudy. *Am J Cardiol* 1993; 71: 1069–73.

174. Rector TS, Kubo SH, Cohn JN. Validity of the Minnesota Living with Heart Failure Questionnaire as a measure of therapeutic response to Enalapril or placebo. *Am J Cardiol* 1993; 71: 1106–7.

175. Reis SE, Holubkov R, Edmundowicz D, et al. Treatment of patients admitted to hospital with congestive heart failure: Specialty-related disparities in practice patterns and outcomes. *J Am Coll Cardiol* 1997; 30: 733–8.

176. Krumholz HM, Parent EM, Tu N, et al. Readmission after hospitalization for congestive heart failure among Medicare beneficiaries. *Arch Intern Med* 1997; 157: 99–104.

177. Burns RB, McCarthy EP, Moskowitz MA, et al. Outcomes for older men and women with congestive heart failure. *J Am Geriatr Soc* 1997; 45: 276–80.

178. Lowe J, Candlish P, Henry D, et al. Management and outcomes of congestive heart failure: A prospective study of hospitalised patients. *MJA* 1998; 168: 115–18.

179. Jaagosild P, Dawson N, Thomas C, et al. Outcomes of acute exacerbation of severe congestive heart failure. *Arch Intern Med* 1998; 158: 1081–9.

180. Rich MW, Beckham V, Wittenberg C, et al. A multidisciplinary intervention to prevent the readmission of elderly patients with congestive heart failure. *New Engl J Med* 1995; 333: 1190–5.

181. Rich MW, Freedland KE. Effect of DRG's on three-month readmission rate of geriatric patients with congestive heart failure. *Am J Publ Hlth* 1988; 78: 680–4.

182. Wolinsky F, Smith D, Stump T, et al. The sequele of hospitalization for congestive heart failure among older adults. *J Am Geriatr Soc* 1997; 45: 558–63.

183. Vinson JM, Rich MW, Sperry JC, et al. Early readmission of elderly patients with congestive heart failure. *J Am Geriatr Soc* 1990; 38: 1290–5.

184. Gooding J, Jette AM. Hospital readmissions among the elderly. *J Am Geriatr Soc* 1985; 33: 595–601.

185. McDermott M, Feinglass J, Lee P, et al. Systolic function, readmission rates, and survival among consecutively hospitalized patients with congestive heart failure. *Am Heart J* 1997; 134: 728–36.

CHAPTER 3

Studies of morbidity and mortality related to heart failure in Scotland

Introduction

As discussed in Chapters 1 and 2, chronic heart failure is a major and growing public health problem in industrialized countries with ageing populations. It is often associated with persistent and debilitating symptoms requiring chronic pharmacotherapy. Periodic episodes of acute clinical deterioration are common and lead to unplanned hospitalization and premature death. Consequently, heart failure imposes a heavy burden on the healthcare system overall, and the hospital sector in particular.[1] Recent reports from the United States[2-4], Scotland[5], Sweden[6], the Netherlands[7], New Zealand[8] and Spain[9] have all described an increase in the number of hospitalizations associated with heart failure. However, with the major exception of a more recent report from the United States relating to the period 1985–95, [3] these reports predominantly describe hospitalization rates that pre-date the widespread use of newer treatments such as angiotensin-converting enzyme (ACE) inhibitors.

As reported previously, Scotland, a country of the United Kingdom with a population of 5.1 million people, has a well-described system for recording details of hospitalizations.[10] This system also permits analyses of hospitalization and survival data on an individual basis. These data were analysed to determine the following:

- Trends in hospitalization related to heart failure in Scotland for the period 1990–96.[11]
- The prognosis for heart failure in people with a first-ever admission with this diagnosis compared with patients with a diagnosis of the most common forms of cancer.[12]
- Whether the prognosis for heart failure has improved since the introduction of more effective therapeutic agents (for example, ACE inhibitors).[13]

Methods

Data source

The Information and Statistics Division of the National Health Service in Scotland collects and collates data on *all* hospital discharges using the Scottish Morbidity Record Scheme.[10] Information from patient case records is used to code diagnoses at the time of hospital discharge. The Ninth and Tenth Revisions of the World Health Organization's International Classification of Diseases (ICD) were used during the period of study (1990–96).[14, 15] The term 'discharge' includes both live discharges and deaths. For those discharged alive, subsequent hospitalizations can be identified for an individual patient using this linked database. These data are also linked to information held by the General Register Office for Scotland, relating to all deaths within the United Kingdom. Consequently, any readmission or death can be identified for a given patient. [10]

Baseline data

Each hospital record provides information concerning individuals' age, sex, date of admission and usual postcode of residence. The postcodes were used to derive the Carstairs-Morris Deprivation index.[14] This index, based on an official Scottish-wide census carried out in 1991, can be used to rank postcodes of residence into five deprivation categories (1 = least deprived, 5 = most deprived) according to levels of employment, living conditions, car ownership and social class.[16] These data also permit identification of those patients who had been admitted to hospital for any other reason during the five years before their admission for heart failure. To consistently obtain a five-year history of prior admission to hospital for each patient, the principal analyses in this study were confined to patients admitted between January 1986 and December 1995. This allowed patients to be followed up for a minimum of one year to the end of the study (31 December 1996).

Trends in hospitalization for heart failure

For the period 1990–96 we identified all hospitalizations in Scotland where heart failure was coded at discharge as either the principal (first position) or secondary diagnosis (second to sixth diagnostic position). This 'episode-based' data set was then analysed to determine the number of men and women who were hospitalized on one or more occasion a year. Using retrospective data (available from 1981) we also identified the annual number of men and women who were experiencing their 'first-ever' hospitalization for heart failure (principal diagnosis).

The following ICD 9 and equivalent ICD 10 codes (introduced in late 1996) were used to determine the presence of heart failure: 402 (hypertensive heart failure), 425.4 (primary cardiomyopathy), 425.5 (alcoholic cardiomyopathy), 425.9 (secondary cardiomyopathy), 428.0 (congestive heart failure), 428.1 (left heart failure and 428.9 (heart failure, unspecified).[14] A recent validation of ICD coding of each hospital discharge in Scotland suggest that diagnostic data are 90% accurate overall.[17]

Is heart failure more malignant than cancer?

The Scottish Cancer Registry also contains these data about individuals, in addition to more specific information about the anatomical site and type of their primary tumour.[18] The four most common sites of cancer registered in Scottish men during 1991 were, in rank order, lung (30%), large bowel (12%), prostate (11%) and bladder (8%). The equivalent figures for women were breast (24%), large bowel (14%), lung (10%) and ovarian cancer (5%).[18]

Socio-demographic and survival data, including sex-specific and age-specific life expectancy, for the whole of the Scottish population (about 5.1 million people) during 1991–96 are contained in the 1991 and 1996 Annual Reports of the Registrar General for Scotland.[19, 20]

Data relating to a first hospitalization for heart failure and acute myocardial infarction in 1991 were obtained from the linked database containing data on hospitalization and survival. Equivalent data about cancer-related diagnoses of interest were obtained from the Scottish Cancer Registry.

All recorded admissions during the year 1991 were screened in order to identify and select all those patients with a hospitalization primarily caused (recorded in the first position for the purpose of ICD9 coding) by the following:

- Heart failure (using the ICD9 codes described above)
- Acute myocardial infarction (ICD9 410)
- Cancer, where the primary tumour was situated in the lung (ICD9 162), large bowel (ICD9 153–4), breast (ICD9 174), prostate (ICD9 185), bladder (ICD9 188) or ovary (ICD9 183).[14]

We then excluded all patients who had a hospital admission for their 'index' condition (recorded in any position for the purpose of ICD9 coding) in the 10 years prior to 1991. For cancer patients a previous admission associated with any malignant neoplasm (ICD9 140–208) also meant they were excluded from analysis.

Survival and loss of expected life years

The Linked Database currently permits reliable analysis of survival data to 31 December 1996. All surviving patients were censored at this time to provide five-year follow-up for every patient. If death from any cause occurred, length of survival was calculated from the date of recorded admission to the date of recorded death.

All individuals who died before their 'expected' age of death (determined by published life-expectancy tables for the age-matched population cohort in 1991[19, 20]) were defined as premature. The number of 'expected' life years lost was also calculated by subtracting actual age at death from 'expected' age of death. Associated loss of expected life years was then calculated as a median (IQR) for each diagnosis and as a rate of expected life years per 1000 population.

Statistical analysis

Sex-specific life tables and Kaplan-Meier survival curves for each condition were constructed from survival data using the actuarial life table method. Comparative, sex-specific and age-specific survival data for the entire Scottish population in 1991 (a census year) were calculated from mid-year population estimates from 1991 to 1996.[19, 20] Multiple logistic regression models were then used to calculate the probability of death within 30 days and, for surviving patients, 31 days to 5 years, adjusting for age and social deprivation. Age was entered into each logistic model as a continuous variable and social deprivation was entered as the original index score from one to five. The six diagnoses were entered into each logistic model as one categorical variable, with heart failure set as the lowest class. For both social deprivation and diagnosis, the lowest class was set at unity. Adjusted odds ratio (OR) and 95% confidence intervals (CI) for myocardial infarction and four types of cancer are therefore relative to that of heart failure. All logistic regression models were subject to the Hosmer-Lemeshow Goodness-of-Fit Test and were accepted as valid if the associated p value was > 0.05. For all analyses SPSS version 9.0 was used.

Improving prognosis in heart failure?

For the purpose of this analysis, a 'first admission' was defined as no admission with heart failure in the past five years. The period of study was 1986 to 1996. Patients with a hospitalization related to heart failure in the previous five years were excluded from this analysis.

Statistical analysis

The Linked Database allowed analysis of survival data for all identified patients until 31 December 1996. All surviving patients were censored at this time point to provide between one and 10 years follow up, depending on the year of the index admission. If death from any cause occurred, survival time was calculated as the time from date of index admission to date of death from any cause. Crude case-fatality rates were calculated for follow-up periods from 30 days to 10 years using the actuarial life table method. This takes account of admission dates and periods of follow up, which differ between patients. Crude case-fatality rates were stratified by age, sex, deprivation category, prior admission ('co-morbidity') and year of first admission for heart failure. Kaplan-Meier analyses were used to determine median survival. For patients admitted to hospital with heart failure, mortality at 30 days was modelled using logistic regression to analyse the independent effects of these factors. As changes in case fatality for men and women seemed to differ in the short term depending on age, the sexes were considered separately in the multivariate analyses. All variables were entered simultaneously into the models. Each model was subject to the Hosmer and Lemeshow Goodness-of-Fit Test and all were statistically non-significant. To examine the independent effect of these factors on survival thereafter, data from patients who survived 30 days or more were entered into Cox's proportional hazard models. Once again, models were performed separately for men and women and all variables were entered simultaneously into the model. The assumption of constant hazard was met for these models. For both multiple logistic regression and Cox's proportional hazards models, age was recoded and entered in ascending order as follows: < 55, 55–64, 65–74, 75–84 and over 84 years of age. Deprivation data were re-entered as the five categories described above. The 2350 patients not assigned a deprivation category were excluded from these analyses. Prior admission categories were entered as either present or absent. Year of admission was coded chronologically from one to 10 (1986–95). For each variable entered into a model, the lowest class was set at unity. Adjusted odds and hazard ratios for the remaining one to nine classes for each variable are therefore relative to that of the lowest class. Significance was accepted at the level of 0.005. All analyses were undertaken using the Statistical Package for Social Scientists (SPSS, Chicago, Illinois 60611).

Results

Trends in hospitalization for heart failure in Scotland, 1990–96: An epidemic that has reached its peak?[11]

Total episodes of hospitalization

Between 1990 and 1996 a total of 158,989 hospital discharges in Scotland were documented where heart failure was coded in any diagnostic position. Overall, women accounted for more hospital discharges (52%) than men, and congestive heart failure was the most common type of heart failure coded (about 90%).

Figures 3.1 (principal diagnosis) and 3.2 (secondary diagnosis) show the sex-specific trends, both in terms of the total number of hospitalizations for heart failure recorded and the number of patients who contributed to these hospitalizations during this period. For both men and women the number of hospitalizations associated with a principal diagnosis of heart failure in 1996 had increased by an additional 744 (16%) and 605 (12%) compared with 1990. However, in women the

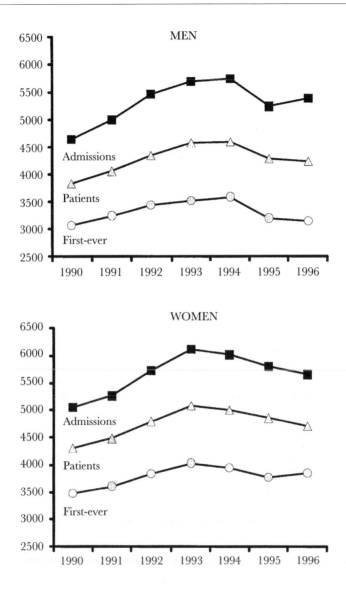

Figure 3.1: Sex-specific trends in the number of hospitalizations for heart failure as the principal diagnosis and the number of patients who contributed to these (including those with a first-ever hospitalization) in Scotland, 1990–96.

highest number of hospitalizations was recorded in 1993 (21% more than in 1990) whereas in men the highest number was in 1994 (24% more than in 1990). During this same period, the number of hospitalizations associated with a secondary diagnosis of heart failure steadily increased in both men (81% more than in 1990)

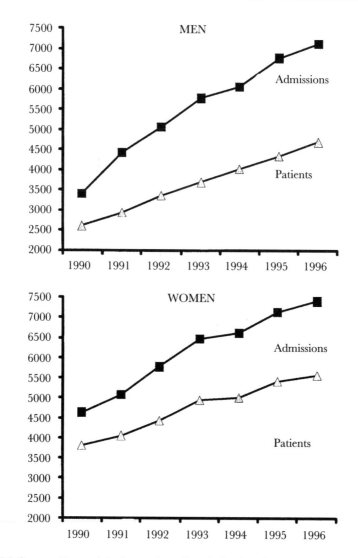

Figure 3.2: Sex-specific trends in the number of hospitalizations for heart failure as a secondary diagnosis and the associated number of patients who contributed to these in Scotland, 1990–96.

and women (60% more than in 1990). In 1996, therefore, there were an additional 3925 (46%) male and 3381 (35%) female hospitalizations recorded with a diagnosis of heart failure (coded in any position) compared with 1990.

Hospitalizations for heart failure as a proportion of all hospital activity in Scotland

Heart failure (coded as the principal diagnosis at discharge) accounted for 1.1% of admissions in both 1990 and 1996. As a secondary coding, heart failure was associated with an additional 0.9% of discharges in 1990 and 1.5% in 1996. Overall, therefore, heart failure, as either a primary or secondary coding, contributed to 2.0% and 2.6% of all discharges from hospital in 1990 and 1996, respectively.

Population rate of hospitalization for heart failure

Table 3.1 shows the population rate of hospitalizations associated with either a principal or secondary diagnosis of heart failure at discharge during 1990–96. While the overall population rate of hospitalization associated with a principal diagnosis of heart failure in both sexes rose slightly in the first four years of this period, in the last two years these rates declined to levels equivalent to those of 1990. However, because of a steady increase in the rate of hospitalizations associated with secondary diagnosis of heart failure, the overall rate of hospitalization for heart failure rose appreciably. This increase was most marked in men, who in 1990 had a lower and by 1996 a higher rate of hospitalization compared with women.

Table 3.1: Annual rate of hospitalization for heart failure per 1000 population in Scotland (1990–96) according to the diagnostic position of heart failure at discharge

	1990	1991	1992	1993	1994	1995	1996
Men							
Principal diagnosis	2.1	2.0	2.2	2.3	2.3	2.1	2.2
Secondary diagnosis	1.4	1.8	2.1	2.3	2.5	2.7	2.9
Any diagnostic position	3.5	3.8	4.3	4.6	4.8	4.8	5.1
Women							
Principal diagnosis	1.9	2.0	2.2	2.4	2.3	2.2	1.9
Secondary diagnosis	1.8	1.9	2.2	2.4	2.5	2.7	2.8
Any diagnostic position	3.7	3.9	4.4	4.8	4.8	4.9	4.7

Age-specific and sex-specific rates of hospitalization

Figure 3.3 shows the age-specific and sex-specific rates of hospitalization as a principal diagnosis of heart failure for men and women aged ≥ 55 years during this period. In all age groups the overall rate of hospitalization related to heart failure (coded in any diagnostic position at discharge) increased appreciably. However, with the exception of men aged ≥ 75 years (who also recorded a modest increase in the number of hospitalizations associated with a principal diagnosis of heart failure) this was almost solely attributable to discharges associated with a secondary diagnosis of heart failure.

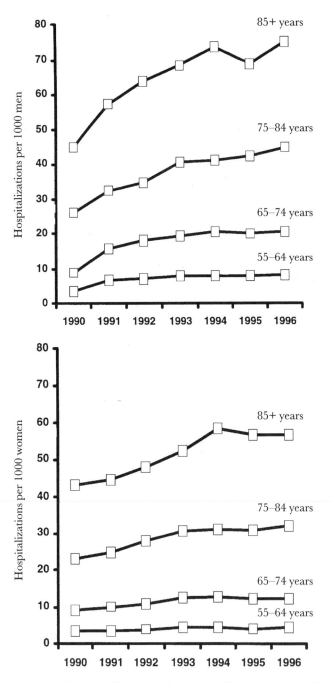

Figure 3.3: Age- and sex-specific population rates of hospitalization in Scotland (1990–96) associated with a principal diagnosis of heart failure.

The average age of men discharged with heart failure (coded in any position) was 71 ± 12 years in 1990 and 71 ± 12 years in 1996 (there was an increase of 0.4 years). The equivalent figures for women were 76 ± 12 years and 77 ± 12 years, respectively (an increase of 0.6 years). Male patients having a 'first-ever' hospitalization for heart failure had an average age in 1990 of 71 ± 12 years and 72 ± 12 years in 1992 (an increase of 0.8 years). In women the equivalent figures for 1990 were 76 ± 11 years and 77 ± 12 years in 1996 – an average age increase of one year. While the proportion of men over 65 years rose from 74% to 78%, the proportion of women over 65 years stayed the same between 1990 and 1996 at 88%.

Ratio of patients to total hospitalizations

Compared with 1990, in 1996 a total of 2201 (414 with a principal diagnosis) more women and 2487 (407 with a principal diagnosis) men were hospitalized – an increase of 21.4% and 26.5% respectively (4.0% and 4.3% respectively for a principal diagnosis of heart failure). Also during this period, the number of men and women with both a principal and a secondary diagnosis hospitalized on more than one occasion during any one year steadily increased (particularly in the latter group) and therefore contributed disproportionately to the total number of hospitalizations. For example, in 1990 13.5% of women and 17% of men recorded multiple hospitalizations compared with 18.5% and 22% respectively in 1996. So, the absolute number of re-hospitalizations a year rose by 53% to 5851 between 1990 and 1996 (representing 23% of all hospitalizations for heart failure in 1996).

Patients admitted for the first time with heart failure

Table 3.2 shows the number of individuals who experienced a first hospitalization associated with a principal diagnosis of heart failure (and no previous hospitalization

Table 3.2: Number of Scottish men and women admitted for the first time with a diagnosis of heart failure (principal) during 1990–96 and their contribution to the overall number of hospitalizations for heart failure

	1990	1991	1992	1993	1994	1995	1996
Men							
First-ever hospitalization	3071	3241	3435	3526	3587	3189	3301
% of all principal diagnoses	66	65	63	62	62	61	61
% of all hospitalizations	44	44	42	43	40	35	38
Women							
First-ever hospitalization	3479	3606	3835	4032	3946	3766	3749
% of all principal diagnoses	69	68	67	66	66	65	66
% of all hospitalizations	43	42	42	40	40	37	39

where heart failure was coded at discharge) between 1990 and 1996 and their relative contribution to the total number of hospitalizations recorded for that year. During this period the absolute number of these 'first-ever' hospitalizations rose until 1993 in women and 1994 in men, but thereafter seemed to decline towards 1990 levels. Overall, the relative contribution of these first-ever hospitalizations to the total number of hospitalizations for heart failure gradually declined throughout 1990–96. The proportion of men and women aged ≥ 65 years who experienced their first-ever hospitalization for heart failure remained constant throughout this period, at 52% and 76% respectively.

Length of stay

In 1990 the length of hospital stay (LOS) varied widely according to the age and type of unit from which a person was discharged and the diagnostic coding position of heart failure at hospital discharge. On average, women, elderly people and those who had been discharged from a geriatric unit had the longest LOS. However, for both sexes and regardless of the diagnostic coding position of heart failure at hospital discharge, median LOS progressively decreased between 1990 and 1996. In 1990 the median LOS for men with a principal diagnosis of heart failure fell from 9 (IQR 5–18) days to 8 (4–16) days in 1996. For women the equivalent figures were 13 (7–27) days in 1990 compared with 10 (5–19) days in 1996. The median LOS for a male and female hospitalized with a secondary diagnosis of heart failure fell from 10 (5–19) and 13 (7–27) days to 8 (3–15) and 10 (5–21) days respectively, between 1990 and 1996. In 1996, therefore, for both sexes, regardless of the diagnostic coding position of heart failure at hospital discharge, the median LOS was broadly the same.

Total days of hospitalization

Despite the overall increase in all hospitalizations associated with a diagnosis of heart failure between 1990 and 1996, the significant falls in LOS resulted in a 12% and 43% decrease in the total number of days of hospitalization a year for men and women respectively. However, the 12,502 male hospitalizations recorded in 1996 still resulted in about 170,000 days of inpatient care (about 68 days/1000 population) and the 13,061 female hospitalizations recorded in the same year resulted in about 230,000 days of inpatient care (about 88 days/1000 population) – see Table 3.3. In 1996, heart failure (as a principal diagnosis) accounted for 1.4% of all inpatient days, 4.7% of internal medicine days and 3.1% of geriatric bed days. The equivalent figures for heart failure coded as a secondary diagnosis were 1.9%, 5.7% and 5.0% respectively. Therefore, heart failure, coded in any diagnostic position, contributed to 10.4% of all internal medicine bed days. Heart failure, as a principal diagnosis, accounted for 4.2% of all internal medicine/

Table 3.3: Days of hospitalization associated with a discharge diagnosis of heart failure in Scotland – 1990 compared with 1996

	1990		1996		1990 vs 1996
	Total days of hospitalization	Days/1000 population	Total days of hospitalization	Days/1000 population	δ in total days per annum
Men					
Principal diagnosis	95,856	36.3	70,413	28.3	−25,443
Secondary diagnosis	93,790	36.6	96,808	38.9	+ 3,018
All diagnostic positions	189,646	71.9	167,221	67.2	−22,425
Women					
Principal diagnosis	169,067	64.1	93,633	35.4	−75,434
Secondary diagnosis	234,985	89.1	136,770	51.8	−98,215
All diagnostic positions	404,052	153.2	230,403	87.2	−173,649

geriatric bed days occupied in Scotland in 1996 (and contributed to 9.6% of these, if a heart failure coding in any position is considered).

In-hospital case fatality

The annual case fatality rate associated with a hospitalization related to heart failure fell steadily for men and women alike and in all age groups during this period. In men, the inpatient case fatality rate associated with a principal diagnosis of heart failure fell slightly from 15.8% in 1990 to 15.2% in 1996, and more substantially from 20.3% to 14.9% in those men discharged with a secondary diagnosis of heart failure. In women, the equivalent case fatality rates fell from 17.5% to 15.6% for a hospitalization associated with a principal diagnosis of heart failure, and from 21% to 15.3% for those discharged with a secondary diagnosis of heart failure. Overall, therefore, in 1996 the case fatality rate in both sexes and irrespective of the diagnostic position of heart failure was 15–16%. However, compared with 1990, in 1996 the total number of deaths in male patients in hospital associated with a principal diagnosis of heart failure had risen by 11% (from 733 to 818 deaths) and deaths associated with any hospitalization related to heart failure rose by 18% (from 1532 to 1878 deaths). In women the total number of deaths in women associated with a principal diagnosis of heart failure remained the same (884 versus 882 deaths), but increased slightly in terms of all hospitalizations related to heart failure.

Is heart failure more malignant than cancer?[12]

Cohort characteristics

In 1991, a total of 16,224 men experienced a 'first-ever' hospitalization for heart failure (n = 3241), AMI (n = 6932) or cancer of the lung, large bowel, prostate or bladder (n = 6051). Similarly, 14,842 women experienced an initial hospitalization for heart failure (n = 3606), AMI (n = 4916), or cancer of the breast, lung, large bowel or ovary (n = 6320). Table 3.4 summarizes the demographic characteristics of this cohort according to their index diagnosis. It also shows the annual population incidence rate for each type of admission.

Overall, there were more first-time admissions for AMI than for heart failure. This difference was greater in men (more than double) than in women (about 40% more). Consistent with data emanating from the UK overall, [18] mainland Europe[21] and the US, [22] lung cancer was the most and second most common form of cancer in men and women. With the exception of acute myocardial infarction (mean age 64 years), male patients were predominantly older than 60 years of age; the age distributions being broadly similar for heart failure and the four types of cancer. Among women, however, there was a clear difference in the age distribution of those admitted with cancer of the breast or ovary (mean age 62–4 years) and the remainder of the cohort (mean age 72–6 years). Although there were

Table 3.4: Demographic profile of all patients admitted to hospital in Scotland in 1991 for the first time with a principal diagnosis of heart failure, myocardial infarction or the four most common types of cancer specific to men and women

Primary cause of a first Admission in 1991	Number of Cases	Percentage of total cases	Mean (SD) age in years	Annual incidence
Men				
Heart failure	3241	47	71 (12)	1.3/1000
Myocardial infarction	6932	59	64 (10)	2.8/1000
Lung cancer	2695	64	69 (10)	0.8/1000
Large bowel cancer	1385	50	69 (11)	0.6/1000
Prostate cancer	1211	100	74 (08)	0.5/1000
Bladder cancer	760	67	69 (11)	0.3/1000
Women				
Heart failure	3606	53	76 (11)	1.4/1000
Myocardial infarction	4916	41	72 (11)	1.9/1000
Breast cancer	2902	100	62 (14)	0.8/1000
Lung cancer	1490	36	70 (10)	0.4/1000
Large bowel cancer	1402	50	72 (12)	0.4/1000
Ovarian cancer	526	100	64 (14)	0.2/1000

about 25% more admissions for heart failure than for breast cancer overall, only 20% of these were among women aged less than 65 years compared with 50% for breast cancer.

Unadjusted survival

For both men and women, lung cancer was associated with the poorest unadjusted survival rate, with a median survival time of 3–4 months and only 5% of patients surviving to 5 years. However, heart failure was associated with the second-poorest unadjusted survival rate, with a median survival time of 16 months and only 25% of men and women surviving to 5 years. Overall, short, medium and longer-term survival rates varied widely according to the index diagnosis (see Figure 3.4). For example, whereas myocardial infarction was associated with a similar (and therefore high) initial mortality rate at 30 days (between

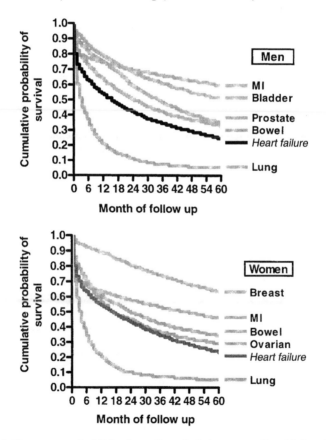

Figure 3.4: Five-year survival following a first admission to any Scottish hospital in 1991 for heart failure, myocardial infarction and the four most common sites of cancer specific to men and women.

20% and 25%), individuals with heart failure fared considerably worse thereafter. Among women, survival following heart failure was broadly equivalent to that following ovarian cancer, whereas breast cancer was associated with twice the survival rate at 5 years (60%).

Adjusted survival relative to heart failure

With the major exception of lung cancer (with about a two-fold and eight-fold increased probability of death in the short term and longer term, respectively), heart failure was associated with the poorest longer-term adjusted survival in men. In women cancer of the breast and cancer of the large bowel were associated with better short-term survival rates in comparison with heart failure: in the longer term, more women survived following breast cancer and an equivalent number survived following bowel cancer or heart failure. Alternatively, cancer of the ovary and lung was associated with poorer adjusted survival rates overall in comparison with heart failure (see Table 3.5). As expected, age was a powerful prognostic factor in both models, each additional decade of age conferring about a four-fold and five-fold increased probability of death within five years for men and women respectively. Figure 3.5 shows the survival rates for the most represented age group

Table 3.5: Probability of survival relative to heart failure in the short and longer term among men and women following a first admission for myocardial infarction and the four most common types of cancer, adjusting for age and deprivation

	Adjusted OR (95% CI) for 30-day mortality	P value	Adjusted OR (95% CI) for 31-day to 5-year mortality	P value
Men				
Heart failure	1.00	–	1.00	–
Myocardial infarction	1.24 (1.11, 1.39)	< 0.001	0.23 (0.21, 0.26)	< 0.001
Bladder cancer	0.19 (0.13, 0.27)	< 0.001	0.54 (0.45, 0.64)	< 0.001
Prostate cancer	0.27 (0.21, 0.34)	< 0.001	0.86 (0.73, 0.98)	< 0.05
Large bowel cancer	0.64 (0.53, 0.77)	< 0.001	0.89 (0.82, 0.97)	< 0.01
Lung cancer	1.86 (1.64, 2.11)	< 0.001	7.64 (6.17, 9.45)	< 0.001
Women				
Heart failure	1.00	–	1.00	–
Myocardial infarction	0.71 (0.67, 0.75)	< 0.001	0.33 (0.30, 0.37)	< 0.001
Breast cancer	0.55 (0.52, 0.59)	< 0.001	0.59 (0.53, 0.64)	< 0.001
Large bowel cancer	0.88 (0.81, 0.94)	< 0.05	0.99 (0.85, 1.19)	NS
Ovarian cancer	1.39 (1.25, 1.55)	< 0.001	2.24 (1.75, 1.69)	< 0.001
Lung cancer	2.81 (2.63, 3.00)	< 0.001	11.6 (8.69, 15.7)	< 0.001

All adjusted odds ratios are relative to that of heart failure.

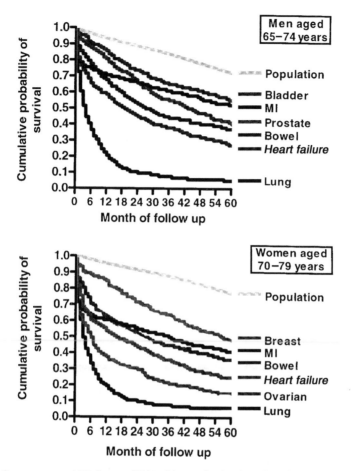

Data for women aged 70–9 years (28% of the total cohort) are based on the following number of patients: heart failure (n = 1167), myocardial infarction (n = 1600) and cancer of the lung (n = 475), breast (n = 441), bowel (n = 369) and ovary (n = 108). Similarly, data for men aged 65–74 years (26% of the total cohort) are based on the following numbers of patients: heart failure (n = 1063), myocardial infarction (n = 2083) and cancer of the lung (n = 1064), bowel (n = 485), prostate (n = 452) and bladder (n = 264).

Figure 3.5: Age-specific probability of survival following a first admission for heart failure, myocardial infarction and the four most common types of cancer specific to men and women relative to the overall population.

for men (65–74 years) and for women (70–9 years) relative to the entire population within that age group. A higher deprivation score was also associated with a two-fold to three-fold higher probability of death relative to the lowest deprivation score.

Loss of expected life years

Table 3.6 shows the total number of deaths associated with each diagnosis, the proportion of which occurred prematurely and the median number of 'expected' life years lost during five-year follow-up. In men, lung cancer was associated with both a large number of premature deaths and a significant number of expected life years lost. Heart failure was also associated with a significant number of expected life years lost (on average 9 years per person), and was associated with more deaths than large bowel, prostate and bladder cancer. In women, despite the fact that proportionately more deaths occurred in those who had already exceeded average life expectancy, heart failure was second only to myocardial infarction in terms of the total number of premature deaths. Both lung cancer and breast cancer, however, by virtue of a greater number of expected life years lost per person, had a greater impact on the population as a whole.

Improving prognosis in heart failure?[13]

Patient characteristics

Between 1986 and 1995 a total of 66,547 patients were admitted to hospital in

Table 3.6: Number of deaths, premature deaths and loss of expected life years for heart failure, AMI and the four most common types of cancer specific to men and women

Index diagnosis in 1991	Total deaths	Premature deaths (%)*	Median (IQR) loss of expected life years/person	Loss of expected life years/1000 population
Men				
Heart failure	2500	1500 (60)	8.7 (4.7, 14.7) years	6.8 years
AMI	2900	1900 (65)	9.7 (4.7, 15.7)	9.4
Lung cancer	2600	1900 (73)	14.4 (5.4, 23.4)	12.3
Large bowel cancer	1000	670 (67)	10.3 (4.3, 17.3)	3.6
Prostate cancer	900	400 (44)	5.6 (3.6, 10.6)	1.2
Bladder cancer	500	230 (46)	6.7 (3.7, 13.7)	0.9
Women				
Heart failure	2800	1200 (43)	6.8 (3.8, 9.8) years	5.1 years
AMI	2800	1400 (50)	7.9 (2.9, 12.9)	6.7
Lung cancer	1400	1100 (79)	13.1 (2.9, 20.1)	6.7
Breast cancer	1300	800 (62)	16.5 (9.5, 23.5)	7.0
Large bowel cancer	1000	520 (52)	10.2 (4.2, 17.2)	3.0
Ovarian cancer	400	300 (75)	14.6 (4.6, 24.6)	2.3

Premature death is defined as any death occurring before an individual's expected age at death (calculated from age-specific life-expectancy data for the Scottish population).

Scotland for the first time with heart failure (principal diagnosis). Consistent with data relating to all admissions related to heart failure, women (n = 35,507) accounted for more than half (53.4%) of this patient cohort. The median age at admission was 78 years in women and 72 years in men. Just over half (53%) of this cohort was aged over 75. Importantly, the median age of women (76.0 years in 1986 compared with 79.0 years in 1995) and men (70.7 years in 1986 compared with 73.0 years in 1995) increased significantly over the period of study (p < 0.0001 for both comparisons).

About one-third of this cohort had a history of a prior hospitalization within five years of the index admission. Acute myocardial infarction (15.1% of the total cohort) and other forms of coronary heart disease (11.1%) were the major reasons for such hospitalization. Significantly, there was a trend over this period for patients to have more prior admissions (other than heart failure). For example, 37% versus 46% of women had at least one prior hospitalization in 1986 and 1995, respectively. The equivalent proportions for men were 42% and 52%, respectively.

Crude case fatality rates

Figure 3.6 shows the short-, medium- and longer-term case-fatality rates for this cohort according to the year of admission. During the whole period of study the crude case fatality rate at 30 days, one year, five years and 10 years in men was 19.4%, 44.0%, 75.0% and 87.2%, respectively. The equivalent rates in women were 20.3%, 44.9%, 76.2% and 89.3%, respectively. Case fatality rates increased

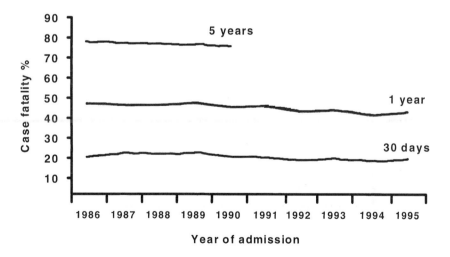

Figure 3.6: Trends in short-, medium- and longer-term case fatality in patients admitted for the first time with a principal diagnosis of heart failure in Scotland (1986–1995).

markedly with age, with one-month and one-year case fatality rates increasing from 10.4% and 24.2% in those aged < 55 years to 25.9% and 58.1% in those aged > 84 years. Median survival over the period of study was 1.5 years in men and 1.4 years in women. For those surviving the initial 30-day period, median survival was 2.5 years in men and 2.4 years in women.

Adjusted case-fatality rates

Multivariate analysis confirmed the powerful effect of age on survival. The adjusted risk of death (30 day to end of follow up) associated with each additional decade of age increased by 1.42-fold in men and 1.38-fold in women. The effect of sex on survival was both modest and complex. There was a highly significant interaction between age and sex, but only for 30-day case fatality. For example, in the short term, young women (aged < 65 years) fared worse than young men, whereas older women (> 65 years) had a better outcome than older men. In the longer term (beyond 30 days), no interaction between age and sex was detected and, overall, women had a lower case fatality than men.

Greater deprivation was associated with a higher short-term case fatality rate (a 26% and 11% increased risk for those men and women in the lowest deprivation category compared with those in the highest). The equivalent risk of longer-term case fatality was increased by 10% in men and 6% in women. In general, a prior admission (regardless of the principal cause) increased the risk of death.

The adjusted odds of 30-day case fatality in men and women for each year of admission with 1986 as the reference year, after adjustment for age, deprivation and prior admission, fell by 26% and 17%, respectively (p < 0.0001 for both comparisons). Figure 3.7 shows the adjusted risk of longer-term case fatality for

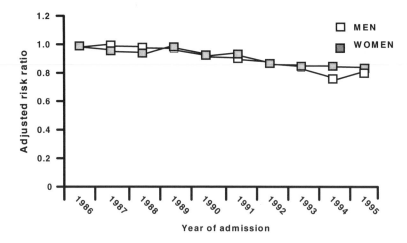

Figure 3.7: Trends in adjusted risk of long-term case fatality in patients admitted for the first time with a principal diagnosis of heart failure in Scotland (1986–1995).

each year of admission. As such, it shows that case fatality rates fell by about 18% in men and 15% in women (p < 0.0001 for both comparisons). These data do, of course, pre-date many important clinical trials[24-27] that have refined the treatment of heart failure and it is possible that case-fatality rates have improved further in the past five years.

Discussion

Trends in hospitalization for heart failure: An epidemic that has reached its peak?

The aim of the first study was to describe recent trends in hospital discharges for heart failure in Scotland, following on from an identical study examining the same subject over the earlier period 1980 to 1990. The original report, by McMurray and colleagues, described a 60% increase in hospitalizations for heart failure between 1980 and 1990 and several subsequent reports confirmed similar findings in other countries.[5]

Comparison with other reports

The present study contrasts considerably with these older reports. Although an increasing incidence and prevalence of heart failure, associated with ageing of the population, has been described, this does not seem to have been reflected in recent trends in hospitalizations for heart failure. Instead, there has been a decline in discharges, with heart failure coded as the primary diagnosis, since about 1993 and a slowing of the rate of increase (or even plateauing) of the number of hospitalizations associated with heart failure coded as a secondary diagnosis. Nevertheless, the number of discharges remains substantially higher than in 1980 (6729 discharges for a first diagnosis of heart failure in 1980 compared with 11,041 in 1996) and heart failure continues to be a significant cause of hospitalization. Heart failure (as a first diagnosis) accounted for about 1.1% of all hospital discharges in 1995 in Scotland compared with 1.7% in the Netherlands in 1993[7] and 1.6% in New Zealand in 1991.[8]

Has the heart failure epidemic reached its peak?

Similar conclusions can be drawn from examination of population rates of discharge, which also plateaued during the time scale of this study. The overall rate is, however, considerably higher than it was in 1980 (male and female rates 1.27 and 1.32 per 1000 of the population in 1980 compared with 2.2 and 1.9/1000 in 1990, for a principal diagnosis of heart failure). This compares with a rate of 2.87 hospitalizations per 1000 population, for men and women, in Sweden in 1995, [23] 1.6/1000 in the Netherlands in 1990[7] and 1.63/1000 in New Zealand in 1988–91.[8]

Analysis of the overall number of individuals admitted is also in keeping with the analysis of episodes and rates. The number of men with heart failure as the primary diagnosis coded at discharge also peaked in 1994 and for women the peak was in 1993 (at 20% and 18% above the numbers in 1990, respectively). However, the number of patients with a discharge related to heart failure coded in *any* position continued to rise between 1990 and 1996 (by 27% in women and 36% in men), although the rate of increase has been much lower since 1993–4 than it was between 1990 and 1993-4. For men the rise was 27% between 1990 and 1993 and 7% between 1993 and 1996. For women these increases were 24% and 3% respectively.

The findings with patients having a 'first-ever' hospitalization with heart failure (see below) were much the same. The number of men peaked in 1994 and the number of women peaked in 1993. The rise in first discharges from 1990 to these peaks was, however, less marked than for episodes of hospitalization or numbers of patients discharged (the increase in men was 15% and in women 16%).

More readmissions

The second new trend we have identified is that of increasing repeat admissions. Whether we look at heart failure as the principal diagnosis at discharge, or heart failure coded in any position, the proportion of patients having multiple hospitalizations is increasing. The absolute number of hospitalizations accounted for by readmissions in a given 12-month period increased by 53% over the period of study. By 1996 these second or subsequent admissions made up almost one-quarter of all hospitalizations related to heart failure. In the 1995 cohort of first-ever admissions with a primary diagnosis of heart failure, 14% were readmitted within three months and 21% within six months. These findings are consistent with a recent report from the Netherlands reporting a 14% readmission rate within six months of discharge.[7]

Declining length of stay

Length of stay (LOS) declined during the period of study, as it did between 1980 and 1990. Indeed, the average LOS declined by a similar amount in the two time periods in question (by 14 days between 1980 and 1990 and by 13 days between 1990 and 1996, in patients with a primary diagnosis of heart failure). This decline is quite impressive given that there has been a slight increase in the age of patients and that there is a strong relationship between older age and longer LOS. The mean LOS is now similar to that in the Netherlands[7] and New Zealand but less than that in Sweden (8.1 days in 1995)[8] and the US.[4] Despite the decline in LOS the absolute burden in bed days remains substantial, with heart failure contributing to almost 10% of internal medicine/geriatric bed days.

Declining case fatality rates

For discharges coding heart failure as the principal diagnosis, inpatient case fatality rates remained static in men, in contrast to the decline between 1980 and 1990.

There was a small fall in case fatality rates in women. This was much less in absolute and relative terms than that noted between 1980 and 1990. The inpatient case fatality rate in men (15.2%) and women (15.6%) with a primary diagnosis of heart failure in 1996 is similar to that reported from the Netherlands in 1993 (15.5% in men and 14.9% in women)[7] but much higher than that recently reported from the US in 1995.[4] Despite the falling case fatality rate and the slowing of the rate of increase in admission rates, the number of deaths from heart failure (coded as the principal diagnosis) in 1996 (2043) was considerably higher than in 1990 (1838) and 1980 (1543).

Comorbidity

We found, as expected, that myocardial ischaemia and infarction were the most commonly coded additional diagnoses at discharge in patients with a hospitalization related to heart failure. Curiously, however, the proportion of patients with such a coding decreased over the period of study. Indeed, in both sexes and regardless of the position in which heart failure was coded (primary or other), there was a decline in the number of additional diagnoses of all types coded between 1990 and 1996. We have no explanation for this phenomenon, although it does not suggest that excessive secondary coding, in general, has accounted for the rise in overall numbers of hospitalizations associated with heart failure (coded in any position).

Limitations

Although the Scottish Morbidity Record dataset is a unique and accurate source of information[10], like any large dataset it has its limitations. The most important of these is the absence of clinically relevant data (for example, indices of systolic and diastolic function and prescribed pharmacotherapy). Moreover, it is difficult to determine what changes over time are products of changes in coding practices and, perhaps, most importantly, changes in admission thresholds. Despite these limitations, the value of having data for a whole country over a prolonged period of time cannot, and should not, be understated.

Conclusions

Clearly, our most interesting and novel finding is that the much predicted 'epidemic' of hospitalizations for heart failure seems to have peaked, at least in Scotland. No matter what measure we looked at, with the exception of hospital discharges associated with a secondary coding of heart failure, there seems to have been a decline in discharges and patients discharged since about 1993–4. This is indeed surprising because an improving survival rate from myocardial infarction and general ageing of the population might be expected to increase the number of incident cases of heart failure. An increasing incidence, coupled with improving survival in patients with established heart failure, might, in turn, be expected to lead to an increased prevalence. If incidence or prevalence is increasing, it does not seem to be associated with either a rising number of 'new' (first-ever) hospitalizations, or overall hospitalizations primarily for heart failure. Of course, an increased incidence or prevalence need not necessarily translate into more hospitalizations, especially if effective treatments are available to reduce admissions. Digoxin, ACE inhibitors and, more recently, beta blockers and spironolactone all do this. In the period of this survey the use of ACE inhibitors increased substantially.

Despite this observation, morbidity related to heart failure remains high and its overall burden on the healthcare system is enormous. Modest declines in admission rates for principal heart failure will do little to lessen this burden given the general ageing of the population. Moreover, the observed rise in admissions for secondary heart failure is extremely concerning, as is the number of recurrent admissions.

Is heart failure more 'malignant' than cancer?

Having established the modern-day burden of heart failure in respect to hospital admissions, we undertook the first population-based study directly comparing survival after heart failure versus cancer. We found that, with the notable exception of lung cancer, a first admission for heart failure is commonly associated with a worse survival rate than an equivalent admission for its common precursor, AMI, and the most common types of cancer. This applies equally to men and women. The five-year survival rate in the almost 7000 men and women (representing 0.14% of the population) initially admitted to a Scottish hospital with heart failure in 1991 was a dismal 25%. Even on an adjusted basis, survival following heart failure was poorer than that after many of the common types of cancer. Significantly, the number of male deaths associated with heart failure was similar to those from lung cancer (about 2500 in each group) and only 400 fewer than those associated with acute myocardial infarction. In women, heart failure, followed closely by myocardial infarction, was associated with the greatest number of deaths overall (about 2700 deaths in each group).

Comparison with other studies

Is it possible to extrapolate these data to other developed countries? Both the one-year and five-year survival rates in this Scottish cohort are equivalent to those of large-scale studies of patients hospitalized for heart failure in both the US[28] and Australia.[29] On an age-adjusted basis they are also broadly equivalent to the community-based Framingham cohorts.[30, 31] Cancer-related incidence and mortality rates in Scotland are consistent with the rates for the UK overall[18] and other northern European countries[21], but are typically higher than those for the US[22] and southern European countries.[21] For those countries such as the US with equivalent survival rates for heart failure, but lower survival rates for cancer, therefore, the relative prognostic importance of heart failure compared with cancer, may be greater than suggested by these data.

The burden of heart failure

Prioritizing levels of healthcare funding is always difficult. However, the overall impact of any disease state has to be measured not only in terms of absolute mortality rates, but the average age of those affected, the disease's effect on quality of life and the type and cost of healthcare resources it typically engenders. Despite relatively fewer deaths and better survival rates overall, we have again shown that deaths related to breast cancer often occur in relatively young women. The level of publicity and healthcare funding that breast cancer currently receives as an important health issue for women is no doubt justified on this basis.[32] However, despite a greater number of women affected and dismal survival rates (in all age groups), heart failure is rarely identified as an important health issue for women. Additional data from the Scottish Cancer Registry[18] suggest that, during the same five-year period, heart failure was associated with a greater number of premature deaths and associated loss of expected life years than cancer of the ovary, cervix and uterus combined. Coupled with the data that link heart failure with poor survival rates overall[30, 31], an increasing number of expensive hospital admissions (as shown above)[11], and poorer self-reported quality of life than any other common medical disorder[33], the current data reinforce the view that heart failure is a major health issue for both men and women.

Benefits of screening and palliative care programmes

In considering the modern-day burden of heart failure, a further comparison with cancer is probably appropriate. In most developed countries, there are specific cancer registries, routine screening programmes (for example, mammography, cervical smears and faecal occult blood tests) and medical care that is closely regulated to ensure optimal treatment and the rapid introduction of new treatments.[18, 21, 22, 32] Moreover, the widespread implementation of formalized palliative care services also ensures that comprehensive care is delivered to patients with end-stage cancer. Despite recent concerns about the effectiveness of breast screening programmes,[34] data from both Europe[21] and the US[22] suggest that this coordinated response to cancer has resulted in significant reductions in the age-adjusted cancer death rate. Another analogy is perhaps hypertension. The severe and deadly form, appropriately named 'malignant hypertension', has all but disappeared as a result of the introduction of hypertension screening programmes and the widespread use of effective anti-hypertensive therapy.[35] As a direct consequence, the prognosis of hypertension has improved and the incidence of hypertensive heart disease has declined dramatically.[35]

Initiatives specific to heart failure

Despite the high prevalence of individuals in the community who have left ventricular systolic dysfunction associated with either untreated symptoms of heart failure, or who are at risk for developing overt heart failure in the future[36], there is a general lack of screening programmes for the early detection and treatment of such individuals.[37] Moreover, pharmacological agents with proven clinical benefit in the treatment of heart failure (for example, angiotensin-converting enzyme inhibitors) are commonly underused.[38] More important, perhaps, is the general lack of specific heart failure registries and coordinated healthcare services once heart failure is diagnosed. As such, there is only limited evidence (as shown above) to suggest that survival related to heart failure has begun to improve in recent years.[13] Both the Framingham[34] and Rochester[39] studies failed to document improved survival rates among individuals with heart failure prior to the widespread introduction of angiotensin-converting enzyme inhibitors. Although we, and others, have recently reported a decline in case fatality rates associated with this type of cohort in recent years (see below), [13, 40] any improvement in this regard is modest when compared with those associated with most types of cancer. In this context, these data support the need for healthcare initiatives that first recognize heart failure as a distinct and significant component of cardiovascular-related morbidity and mortality, and second afford it the same type of commitment and healthcare resources usually reserved for high-profile disease states. Nurse-led, comprehensive management programmes, for example, have been shown to minimize readmissions and prolong survival in patients with heart failure (see Chapters 5 and 6), [41] but they are underfunded. Such a response needs to be taken as a matter of urgency, especially if, as many people suspect, heart failure reaches 'epidemic' proportions within the next 20 years.[42]

Limitations

As with any study of this type there are a number of limitations that require comment. First, we had to rely on discharge coding to identify the study cohort. Although internal validation studies of the Scottish Morbidity Record Scheme have proved these data to be quite accurate[17] and hospitalization for heart failure is usually associated with more definitive investigation and treatment[43], the diagnostic accuracy and overall quality of data may vary on an institutional basis. Moreover, we do not know what proportion of individuals with a diagnosis of heart failure had left ventricular systolic dysfunction. Heart failure patients with normal systolic function probably have better survival rates than those with depressed function.[44] We have therefore described the survival rate for a mixture of such patients, as have the Framingham[30, 31], Rochester[39] and other studies of this type. We have also only studied patients hospitalized for heart failure who potentially represent the severe end of the spectrum of this syndrome. However, community surveys show that most patients with heart failure are admitted to hospital within two years of identification.[44] Finally, we also have no data concerning causality of subsequent death. This is always problematic because heart failure is commonly omitted from the death certificate as a contributory cause of death.[45]

Conclusions

We have taken the opportunity afforded by the relatively unique linked database in Scotland to directly compare cancer-related survival with that of heart failure. These data show that patients admitted to hospital with a diagnosis of cancer often survive longer than those with a diagnosis of heart failure. As such, for both men and women, heart failure that is severe enough to require hospitalization is more 'malignant' than many of the common types of cancer. On this basis alone, it represents a serious health issue that deserves a more concerted and coordinated response to optimize its early detection and treatment.[35]

The key question, of course, is whether case fatality rates related to heart failure have declined appreciably since 1991. We certainly know that, with the notable exception of lung cancer, mortality rates related to cancer are improving with better treatment. Has the management of heart failure kept pace with that of cancer, or has the disparity become greater?

Improving prognosis in heart failure?

Given the enormous amount of energy directed towards achieving better health outcomes in heart failure, it is important to know whether (a) the clinical trial results are relevant to the general population and (b) whether therapeutic advances have indeed made an impact in relation to the poor prognosis associated with heart failure. In this context, using unique data from a whole population of a single country (Scotland) in our third study, we have confirmed that unselected, and therefore more representative, patients with heart failure are markedly different from those typically enrolled in clinical trials. Overall they are older and more likely to be female.[46] Not surprisingly, perhaps, these data show that the prognosis for patients admitted to hospital with heart failure is worse than that indicated by clinical trials. Survival rates are dismal with an approximate case fatality rate of 20% at 30 days, rising to more than 75% within five years. So, median survival is about 18 months.

Comparison with other studies

How do our findings compare with those of other population-based studies? Overall, our findings are remarkably similar to those reported by the Framingham investigators. For example, median survival in the Framingham population was 1.66 years in men and 3.2 years in women. Moreover, they also reported better survival in patients with a presumed coronary aetiology (although, interestingly, this finding contrasts with some clinical trials).[30, 31] The Rochester Epidemiology investigators described the prognosis in 107 patients presenting to associated hospitals with new onset heart failure in 1981, and 141 patients presenting in 1991. As with the current report, they found that the age of heart failure increased over time – the mean age of patients in 1981 was 75 years, rising to 77 years in 1991.[39]

Improving survival?

Are case fatality rates associated with heart failure actually improving? Previous reports, including the Rochester Epidemiology Study, have suggested that both crude and adjusted case fatality rates have remained stable over time.[39] However, studies such as the Rochester Study examined case fatality rates before the widespread introduction of ACE inhibitors in particular. As suggested earlier, it is difficult to extrapolate the impact of ACE inhibitors and beta blockers on case fatality rates in the 'real world' when they have been tested largely in middle-aged men.[47] Importantly, we have been able to examine case fatality rates in a typically older patient population over a prolonged period of time during which time treatment of heart failure began to change dramatically with the introduction of ACE inhibitors.

The second major finding in our study is that case fatality in patients admitted to hospital with heart failure has been falling over the past decade. Adjusted short-term case fatality has fallen by about 20–25% and longer-term case fatality by 15–20%. Thus median life expectancy has increased by almost half a year. This is a quite different finding from that reported by the Framingham investigators in 1993[30, 31], looking at patients developing heart failure in the period 1948–88, and the Rochester investigators in the period 1981–91.[39] As noted above, in both of these studies no temporal change in prognosis was identified. It is possible that the observed decline in case fatality rates in Scotland reflects a true improvement in survival, consequent on better treatment. However, given that clinical trial cohorts are inherently different from the true population of patients with heart failure, this observation must remain speculative until 'effective' agents are tested in older cohorts with roughly equal numbers of men and women. Although changing admission thresholds may account for our observations, we have no evidence to support this.

Limitations

Although these data provide some evidence that the prognosis in heart failure is improving, our inability to specifically account for factors that have a major bearing on survival (for example, extent of left ventricular systolic dysfunction and drug treatment during and after hospitalization) represents an important limitation when interpreting this study. Apart from this major limitation, common to any study of this type, it should be remembered that we examined patients with heart failure who were admitted to hospital. Arguably, these are patients at the more severe end of the spectrum of heart failure. However, community surveys show that most patients with heart failure have been admitted to hospital, the majority within two years of identification.[43]

Conclusions

Despite a number of limitations, these data provide an important insight into the impact of modern-day treatment of heart failure. In brief, the prognosis of patients admitted to hospital for the first time with a diagnosis of heart failure is very poor indeed. Although there is cause for some optimism (owing to a modest increase in survival), there is still much room for improvement.[47, 48] There is little chance, for example, that survival rates following heart failure have improved beyond the survival rate for the most common forms of cancer.

Summary

In a series of three studies *we** (see note below)[11–13] reconfirmed previous reports suggesting that heart failure is a major burden on the healthcare system and is associated with a particularly poor prognosis. For example, in examining recent trends in hospitalization for heart failure within a whole population, we have confirmed that this index of the morbidity relating to heart failure continues to rise. Similarly, we have confirmed, once again in a whole population, that heart failure is often associated with a prognosis similar to, or even worse than, many forms of cancer. The overall picture, however, is not all that pessimistic. In examining trends in hospitalization we have discovered some evidence that this modern-day epidemic may have reached its peak. Moreover, we have shown that the prognostic outlook for patients hospitalized with heart failure is actually improving – albeit modestly. Clearly, we await corroborating evidence from other countries before claiming that these data suggest a 'new horizon' for heart failure. It is worth noting that in Chapter 7 we provide direct evidence that these Scottish data do have true relevance to other developed countries.

For the present, in the absence of any dramatic developments in preventing and treating heart failure, the healthcare system has to respond to the heart failure epidemic by understanding the reason for the high morbidity and mortality rates that often accompany this truly 'malignant' syndrome. The next few chapters describe some of the reasons for poor health outcomes in heart failure and our efforts to develop a new strategy that will respond to the deficiencies in the healthcare system and provide hope for heart failure patients.

---

*It is important, at this point, to acknowledge that the 'we' in this chapter refers to not only me but includes the combined wisdom and efforts of three of the most influential investigators in the field of cardiological epidemiology – Dr Kate MacIntyre and Professor John McMurray from the University of Glasgow and Professor Simon Capewell from the University of Liverpool, United Kingdom.

References

1. Murray J, Hart W, Rhodes G. An evaluation of the cost of heart failure to the National Health Service in the UK. *Br J Med Econ* 1993; 6: 91–8.
2. Gillum R. Epidemiology of heart failure in the United States. *Am Heart J* 1993; 126: 1042–6.
3. Ghali J, Cooper R, Ford E. Trends in hospitalization rates for heart failure in the United States, 1973–1986. *Arch Intern Med* 1990; 150: 769–73.
4. Haldeman GA, Croft JB, Giles WH, et al. Hospitalization of patients with heart failure: National hospital discharge survey 1985–95. *Am Heart J* 1999; 137: 352–60.
5. McMurray J, McDonagh T, Morrison CE, et al. Trends in hospitalization for heart failure in Scotland 1980–1990. *Eur Heart J* 1993; 14: 1158–62.
6. Eriksson H, Wilhelmsen L, Caidahl K, et al. Epidemiology and prognosis of heart failure. *Zeitschrift für Kardiologie* 1991; 80: 1–6.
7. Reitsma JB, Mosterd A, de Craen AJM, et al. Increase in hospital admission rates for heart failure in the Netherlands, 1980–1993. *Heart* 1996; 76: 388–92.
8. Doughty R, Yee T, Sharpe N, et al. Hospital admissions and deaths due to congestive heart failure in New Zealand, 1988–91. *NZ Med J* 1995; 108: 473–5.
9. Rodriguez-Artalejo F, Guallar-Castillon P, Banegas Banegas JR, et al. Trends in hospitalization and mortality for heart failure in Spain, 1980–1993. *Eur Heart J* 1997; 18: 1771–9.
10. Kendrick S, Clarke J. The Scottish record linkage system. *Health Bull* 1993; 51: 72–9.
11. Stewart S, MacIntyre K, McCleod MC, et al. Trends in heart failure hospitalisations in Scotland, 1990–1996: An epidemic that has reached its peak? *Eur Heart J* 2000; 22: 209–17.
12. Stewart S, MacIntyre K, Hole DA, et al. More malignant than cancer? Five-year survival following a first admission for heart failure in Scotland. *Eur J Heart Fail* 2001; 3: 315–22.
13. MacIntyre K, Capewell S, Stewart S, et al. Evidence of improving prognosis in heart failure: Trends in case-fatality in 66, 547 patients hospitalised between 1986 and 1995. *Circulation* 2000; 102: 1126–31.
14. World Health Organization. *Manual of the International Statistical Classification of Diseases, Injuries and Causes of Death, 9th Revision.* Geneva: WHO, 1977.
15. World Health Organization. *Manual of the International Statistical Classification of Diseases, Injuries and Causes of Death, 10th Revision.* Geneva: WHO, 1996.
16. Carstairs V, Morris R. *Deprivation and Health in Scotland.* Aberdeen: Aberdeen University Press, 1991.
17. Harley K, Jones C. Quality of Scottish morbidity record (SMR) data. *Health Bull* 1996; 54: 410–17.
18. Black RJ, Sharp L, Kendrick SW. *Trends in Cancer Survival in Scotland 1968–1990.* Edinburgh: Information and Statistics Division, 1993.
19. General Register Office for Scotland. *Registrar General's Annual Report for 1991.* Edinburgh: HMSO, 1992.
20. General Register Office for Scotland. *Registrar General's Annual Report for 1996.* Edinburgh: Stationery Office, 1997.
21. Esteve J, Kricker A, Ferlay J, et al., eds. *Facts and Figures of Cancer in the European Community.* Lyon: International Agency for Research on Cancer Scientific Publications, 1993.
22. Wingo PA, Ries LA, Giovino GA, et al. Annual report to the nation on the status of cancer, 1973–1996, with a special section on lung cancer and tobacco smoking. *J Natl Cancer Inst* 1999; 91: 675–90.

23. Rydén-Bergsten T, Andersson F. The health care costs of heart failure in Sweden. *J Intern Med* 1999: 246; 275–84.

24. The Digitalis Investigation Group. The effect of digoxin on mortality and morbidity in patients with heart failure. *N Engl J Med* 1997; 336: 525–33.

25. Packer M, Poole-Wilson PA, Armstrong PW, et al. Comparative effects of low and high doses of the angiotensin converting enzyme inhibitor, lisinopril, on morbidity and mortality in chronic heart failure. *Circulation* 1999; 100: 2312–18.

26. MERIT Investigators. Effect of metoprolol CR/XL in chronic heart failure: Metoprolol CR/XL Randomised Intervention Trial in Congestive Heart Failure (Merit-HF). *Lancet* 1999; 353: 2001–7.

27. Pitt B, Zannad F, Remme WJ, et al. The effect of spironolactone on morbidity and mortality in patients with severe heart failure. Randomized Aldactone Evaluation Study Investigators. *N Engl J Med* 1999; 341: 709–17.

28. Jaagosild P, Dawson N, Thomas C, et al. Outcomes of acute exacerbation of severe congestive heart failure. *Arch Intern Med* 1998; 158: 1081–9.

29. Lowe J, Candlish P, Henry D, et al. Management and outcomes of congestive heart failure: A prospective study of hospitalised patients. *MJA* 1998; 168: 115–18.

30. McKee PA, Castelli WP, McNamara PM, et al. The natural history of congestive heart failure: The Framingham study. *N Engl J Med* 1971; 285: 1441–6.

31. Ho KK, Anderson K, Kannel WB, et al. Survival after the onset of congestive heart failure in Framingham Heart Study subjects. *Circulation* 1993; 88: 107–15.

32. Scottish Intercollegiate Guidelines Network – Scottish Cancer Therapy Network. *Breast Cancer in Women*. Edinburgh: Royal College of Physicians, 1998.

33. Stewart AL, Greenfield S, Hays RD, et al. Functional status and well-being of patients with chronic conditions. Results from the Medical Outcomes Study. *JAMA* 1989; 262: 907–13.

34. PC Gøtzsche, O Olsen. Is screening for breast cancer with mammography justifiable? *Lancet* 2000; 335: 129–34.

35. World Health Organization. *Hypertension Control*. Report of a WHO Expert Committee. *WHO Tech Rep Ser* 1996; 862: 1–83.

36. McDonagh TA, Morrison CE, Lawrence A, et al. Symptomatic and asymptomatic left-ventricular systolic dysfunction in an urban population. *Lancet* 1997; 350: 829–33.

37. McMurray JV, McDonagh TA, Davie AP, et al. Should we screen for asymptomatic left ventricular dysfunction to prevent heart failure? *Eur Heart J* 1998; 19: 842–6.

38. Luzier A, Forrest A, Adelman M, et al. Impact of angiotensin-converting enzyme inhibitor underdosing on rehospitalization rates in congestive heart failure. *Am J Cardiol* 1998; 82: 465–9.

39. Senni M, Tribouilloy CM, Rodeheffer RJ, et al. Congestive heart failure in the community: Trends in incidence and survival in a 10-year period. *Arch Intern Med* 1999; 159: 29–34.

40. Cleland JG, Gemmel I, Khand A, et al. Is the prognosis of heart failure improving? *Eur J Heart Fail* 1999; 1: 229–41.

41. Stewart S, Marley JE, Horowitz JD. Effects of a multidisciplinary, home-based intervention on unplanned readmissions and survival among patients with congestive heart failure: A randomised controlled study. *Lancet* 1999; 354: 1077–83.

42. Bonneux L, Barendregt MA, Meeter K, et al. Estimating clinical morbidity due to

ischemic heart disease and congestive heart failure: The future rise of heart failure. *Am J Public Health* 1994; 84: 20–8.

43. Clarke KW, Gray D, Hampton JR. Evidence of inadequate investigation and treatment of patients with heart failure. *Br Heart J* 1994; 71: 584–7.

44. Vasan RS, Larson MG, Benjamin EJ, et al. Congestive heart failure in subjects with normal versus reduced left ventricular ejection fraction – Prevalence and mortality in a population-based cohort. *J Am Coll Cardiol* 1999; 33: 1948–55.

45. Murdoch DR, Love MP, Robb SD, et al. Importance of heart failure as a cause of death. *Eur Heart J* 1998; 19: 1829–35.

46. Petrie M, Berry C, Stewart S, et al. Failing ageing hearts. *Eur Heart J*, 2001; 22: 1978–90.

47. Parmley WW. Heart failure awareness week: February 14–21. *J Am Coll Cardiol* 2000; 35: 534.

48. Konstam MA. Progress in heart failure management? Lessons from the real world. *Circulation* 2000; 102: 1076.

CHAPTER 4

Determinants of therapeutic efficacy in chronic heart failure: Achieving optimal health outcomes

Introduction

As shown in Chapter 3, which described studies examining the burden of heart failure in the whole population of Scotland, both in terms of morbidity and mortality, there are clearly some important and often costly limitations with respect to the therapeutic impact of the pharmacological agents used to treat chronic heart failure, even under the controlled circumstances of clinical trials. In this context there are a number of factors that are relevant to the full spectrum of cardiac disease states and their therapeutic management that have the potential to influence subsequent health outcomes. Such factors include:

1. ***The diagnostic process.*** There is an obvious need in any clinical situation to accurately determine the underlying pathophysiology and extent of risk of morbidity and mortality in order to administer appropriate treatment. For example, identifying S-T segment depression on the initial ECG of patients admitted to a coronary care unit with a provisional diagnosis of intermediate coronary syndrome indicates high or possibly very high risk of subsequent MI and/or death requiring initiation of maximal treatment and early surgical intervention.[1] Conversely, an accurate diagnosis is important to avoid use of inappropriate treatment such as the application of a non-dihydropyridine calcium antagonist in the context of a patient with an acute coronary syndrome and concurrent severe left ventricular dysfunction.[2]

2. ***Nature of the disease state: Acute versus chronic/benign versus malignant.*** Although suboptimal management of chronic exertional angina will predictably result in recurrent but relatively benign anginal symptoms that resolve at rest, suboptimal management of acute coronary syndrome may result in permanent left ventricular systolic dysfunction and/or premature death secondary to the development of an AMI. Similarly, individuals with severe congestive heart failure often have labile clinical symptoms and are at greater risk of developing acute pulmonary oedema requiring hospitalization if they do not receive appropriate treatment.

3. ***Qualities of the therapeutic modality.*** By their very nature, most of the 'potent' pharmacological agents used in the management of cardiac disease states may be associated with serious adverse effects. As such, there is often a fine line between the benefits and risks conferred by an individual pharmacological agent. In this respect any anticipated therapeutic effect may be attenuated by extraneous factors – for example, the development of digoxin toxicity secondary to a combination of underlying ACE inhibition and a lower than normal fluid intake (leading to renal dysfunction). Similarly, the benefit to risk ratio may depend entirely on the particular dosage of the drug used. For example, although higher doses of glycoprotein IIb/IIIa receptor blockers offer some clinical benefits in comparison to conventional treatment for the management of acute coronary syndromes, they are also associated with higher rates of bleeding.[3]

4. ***Delivery of the therapeutic modality.*** In many cases the mode of delivery of a drug will determine the outcome of treatment. For example, intravenous nitrates are much more effective in the management of acute coronary syndromes than oral forms of the drug.[4] Similarly, the development of subcutaneous preparations of low molecular weight heparin and its use beyond the initial treatment of acute coronary syndrome has been driven in part by the limitations of unfractionated heparin, which usually requires a continuous infusion to maintain adequate anti-coagulation (and regular measurement of activated pro-thrombin times) and is therefore less practical as a post-discharge treatment[5], despite the continuing risk of thrombus formation following initial treatment.[6]

5. ***Stimuli for recurrence of acute events.*** As discussed above, the inherent instability of any disease state and the threshold required to precipitate an acute recurrence will often determine the therapeutic effectiveness of pharmacological treatment. Patients with severe congestive heart failure, for example, often tread a fine line between adequate hydration and fluid overload precipitating acute pulmonary oedema with factors such as incremental myocardial ischaemia, arrhythmias or respiratory infection likely to result in clinical instability.

There are many factors, therefore, that can determine the therapeutic outcome in the management of cardiac disease states. In this context, chronic congestive heart failure represents a disease state in which the potential for a suboptimal outcome, especially for the individual, is high.

Potential determinants of therapeutic response in congestive heart failure

In this context, there are a number of previously identified and often interrelated determinants of therapeutic response in chronic cardiac disease states in general that have particular significance to the longer-term management of chronic heart failure. These include:

1. ***Adequacy of treatment.*** A number of studies have shown that despite the availability of clear clinical guidelines[7–9], a considerable proportion of patients with chronic heart failure often receive suboptimal treatment, especially if they are treated by a non-specialist.[10–12]

2. ***Adverse effects of pharmacological treatment.*** In patients with chronic disease states, there is evidence that much long-term morbidity and perhaps mortality may be related to suboptimal use and/or monitoring of medications. For example, about 2–15% of hospital admissions (depending on the criteria used) in such patients have been attributed to adverse effects of prescribed medications.[13–21]

3. ***Non-adherence to treatment.*** Studies that examine rates of adherence to treatment among older individuals in particular with chronic disease states consistently show that about half of these individuals significantly deviate from their prescribed treatment regimen.[21–22]

4. ***Inadequate in-hospital and post-discharge care.*** Intuitively, it would seem to be safe to assume that increased medical supervision begets better health outcomes, especially among individuals with labile disease states such as severe chronic heart failure and chronic airways limitation. However, a recent controlled study of increased primary care contact with physicians actually suggested poorer health outcomes overall.[23] Despite this study, however, a number of other studies have shown that the extent of post-hospitalization follow-up care and the ability or willingness of patients to access such care have been identified as important determinants of health outcomes among the chronically ill.[23–33]

The challenge of the current management of chronic heart failure, therefore, is to recognize the impact of these factors and to design cost-effective strategies that adequately identify and address them and therefore provide (at least to the current standard) optimal management.

In summary, it is clear that the degree to which either suboptimal management or an incomplete response to a pharmacological regimen will impact on an individual's health will undoubtedly vary, depending on the stability and severity of the disease state and the relative safety of the medication regimen.

Practical considerations for introducing effective strategies to optimize the management of chronic heart failure

In lieu of the next major advance in the pharmacological (or surgical) treatment of chronic heart failure, there is clearly a need to develop (if possible) non-pharmacological strategies that maximize the therapeutic impact of the current therapeutic armoury available to treat older patients.[34, 35] In this respect, a strategy that incorporates the following (and inherently logical) steps seems to be warranted:

1. Identify those individuals with chronic heart failure who are most at risk of experiencing relatively poorer health outcomes (poor quality of life, recurrent hospitalization and/or premature death) and are therefore potential 'therapeutic underachievers'.
2. Identify what deficiencies in the current management of chronic disease states, and chronic heart failure in particular, contribute to the existence of 'therapeutic underachievers' and poorer than expected health outcomes in general.
3. Design and test innovative strategies that simultaneously target potential therapeutic underachievers and the preventable factors (relating to both the individual and their overall healthcare management) that contribute to poorer health outcomes.

Considering the disproportionate contribution of hospital costs to the overall expenditure related to management of heart failure (in most studies this is 60–80% of total costs)[36], any strategy that significantly reduces this component of healthcare use is likely to prove cost-effective.[37] It might also be anticipated that such benefits on healthcare costs would be associated with a parallel improvement in quality of life among the large number of patients with chronic heart failure.

Identifying 'therapeutic underachievers' in the population with chronic heart failure

As discussed in previous chapters, a number of epidemiological studies, using a variety of criteria to define and identify chronic heart failure in the overall population, have examined the prognostic implications and use of healthcare facilities associated with the development of heart failure. Although such studies provide an important insight into the overall survival prospects of individuals with heart failure, they give limited information for determining the subset(s) of individuals with chronic heart failure who require relatively greater use of healthcare resources and/or have poorer survival prospects. These studies do, however, clearly indicate that a large proportion of patients with heart failure are relatively stable and avoid regular institutional care and that hospitalized patients are therefore a relatively small subset of the overall population with heart failure.

It would come as no surprise to clinicians that one hospital admission predisposes towards more hospital admissions among the chronically ill. In this respect, prior hospital use is probably the most consistent and robust predictor of future hospital use among chronically ill patients.[25, 28, 33] Although it would be ideal to prevent all patients with chronic heart failure from experiencing even one hospital admission, achieving this objective would prove problematic.

Widespread early use of appropriate pharmacotherapy (including ACE inhibition) among individuals with asymptomatic left ventricular systolic dysfunction may provide some benefit in this regard.[38, 39] The use of potentially sensitive biochemical markers of left ventricular systolic dysfunction (such as atrial and brain natriuretic peptide) to screen for such patients is one example of this kind of approach that is yet to be proved practical and cost-effective.[40] Perhaps the relative cases for intervention strategies in heart failure during asymptomatic versus symptomatic stages are best summarized by the two arms of the SOLVD study.[41, 42] Whereas treatment of asymptomatic patients delayed onset of symptoms, its effect on mortality was equivocal. Treatment of symptomatic individuals with an identical regimen had a far larger impact on morbidity and mortality. At this stage, therefore, the most cost-effective method for identifying patients at risk of hospitalization is probably to 'capture' them either on the threshold of an admission (in the emergency room), during a hospital admission or following hospitalization in the clinic setting.

Studies of hospital-based care and chronic congestive heart failure

A number of studies have specifically examined the clinical and demographic characteristics and health outcomes of patients with heart failure who require hospital-based care.[43–57] As such, they are undoubtedly biased in that such patients are more likely to have severe heart failure and receive more extensive and intensive specialist care (whether it be as an inpatient or as an outpatient) than most patients with heart failure.[58] Any interpretation of these studies should, therefore, recognize the reciprocal problem of extrapolating treatment response and health outcomes in this subset of patients to the overall heart failure population. However, it is on this basis that they are most useful in prospectively identifying the most problematic patients, as they examine those patients who have already 'revealed' themselves as relatively higher risk in comparison with the majority of patients who avoid prolonged contact with large healthcare institutions, and differentiate these patients on the basis of their response/non-responsiveness to what should be optimal and intensive treatment.

Those studies that specifically examine the interaction between hospital-based care and heart failure (as opposed to those that simply examine hospitalization rates – for example, the studies described in Chapter 3) can be differentiated on the basis of the inclusion criteria used to select their patient population. In this respect, it is important to note that there are generally three types of heart failure cohorts described in the literature:

1. Relatively younger patients who are being managed through a tertiary referral centre with possible intervention with heart transplantation; such patients

constitute a small minority who generally have far less co-morbidity in comparison with older (and more typical) patients with heart failure. [43–45, 59]

2. Patients who may or may not have been hospitalized and are being managed through hospital outpatient clinics.[45–48]

3. Hospitalized patients who have been selected primarily on the basis of presence of heart failure and therefore tend to be older and more representative of the overall population of patients with heart failure. [49–57]

It is the latter type of study that offers the most useful data for identifying patients with chronic heart failure who would benefit in the short/medium term from adjunctive interventions designed to optimize therapeutic outcomes. Importantly, many of these studies include patients hospitalized because of heart failure and those in whom this was an associated diagnosis. In some cases, of course (such as occurrence of pneumonia in patients with heart failure), the distinction might be nebulous and indeed the study described in Chapter 3 suggests that a diagnosis of heart failure is the most important determinant of outcome (including length of stay, readmission and mortality) in such patients. Although these studies vary in location, inclusion criteria, size of cohort and duration of follow-up, the profile and outcomes of hospitalized cohorts studied highlight a number of factors and issues relevant to identifying 'high-risk' patients with chronic heart failure. The most important of these is that relatively unselected patients with heart failure who require acute hospitalization bear little resemblance (both in terms of baseline demographic and clinical characteristics and subsequent health outcomes) to most patients with heart failure included in contemporary clinical trials – this, of course, was evident in our study examining potential improvements in the prognosis for patients with heart failure. This phenomenon is not confined to heart failure but is also evident in the context of myocardial infarction.[60] The most obvious difference in this regard is the age of patients and the inherent gender imbalance among patients in clinical trials.[61] With very few exceptions, including the ELITE Study where patients with heart failure aged ≥ 65 years[62] were specifically chosen and the Prime II Study[63] where the inclusion criteria (unlike in most clinical trials) required hospitalization within two months of study entry, most patients in clinical trials are aged ≤ 65 years.[35] The age differential between patients in clinical trials and hospitalized cohorts of patients with heart failure may partially explain the marked difference in the proportion of females included for study; in most hospital-based studies, female patients predominated (between 50 and 60%) and, when specifically examined, were shown to be older than their male counterparts.[35] This may also reflect the fact that among older and female patients with heart failure there is likely to be a substantial proportion of individuals with mainly diastolic failure[35, 64] and most of the contemporary clinical trial patients have been selected on the basis of documented moderate to severe left ventricular systolic dysfunction. Although selecting patient cohorts on the basis of this parameter allows for more homogeneous cohort characteristics (including treatment and possibly gender), it is likely that the estimated 50% of older patients who have normal left ventricular systolic function will be excluded.[35, 64] Such patients are more likely to exhibit diastolic dysfunction secondary to more prolonged exposure to chronic hypertension.[65] However, among older cohorts of hospitalized patients with heart failure in whom formal measurement of systolic function has been performed, relatively greater diastolic dysfunction has not been correlated with greater hospital use or mortality. This may reflect the fact that older individuals with intact left ventricular systolic function do as poorly as those with some dysfunction[52], or that the commonly used parameter of left ventricular ejection fraction (LVEF) is subject to too much variability according to clinical status (for example, in the presence of paroxysmal atrial fibrillation[66, 67] or fluctuating coronary blood flow[68]) and/or estimative accuracy.[69] On balance, it would seem that although older patients with severe systolic dysfunction are at greater risk of dying in the six to 12 months following acute hospitalization, [53] there is little evidence that, even when accounting for reduced periods of follow-up, such patients use hospitals more than patients with relatively intact systolic function.

Although the relative importance of systolic versus diastolic dysfunction as predictors of subsequent morbidity and mortality in hospitalized patients remains uncertain, it seems that the extent of functional impairment and/or hospitalization (especially that associated with chronic heart failure) are important indicators of outcome in such patients.[70, 71] Overall, these data suggest that heart failure patients' functional status is more important than their left ventricular ejection fraction when trying to predict outcome, especially when examining their risk of subsequent hospitalization. Studies of hospitalized patients with heart failure, not surprisingly, show that most patients have functional impairment corresponding to New York Heart Association Class III or IV on admission. Furthermore, they consistently show that up to 20% of hospitalized patients experience repeated admissions to hospital during a short period of time (for example six months).[53–57] Despite the paucity of data relating to prospective determination of frequent, recurrent admissions among patients with heart failure, it is clear that such patients have a less favourable outcome than those who avoid hospitalization.[54] The high frequency of readmission among patients with chronic heart failure is not simply as a result of acute episodes of heart failure, in fact most readmissions among the studied cohorts were for conditions other than heart failure, representing up to two-thirds of admissions. This observation was supported by the study data described in Chapter 3. Indeed these latest data suggest that the future burden of heart failure will be predominantly as a secondary diagnosis complicating treatment. Where data are available, it is clear that concurrent, chronic co-morbid conditions including ischaemic heart disease, atrial fibrillation, diabetes, chronic airways disease and renal insufficiency, which are both debilitating in themselves and likely to confound and complicate the management of heart failure, are often prevalent in these patients.[72]

It is no surprise, therefore, that those studies that specifically examine the outcomes of predominantly older and more gender-balanced cohorts of patients with heart failure, who have had at least one episode of clinical instability requiring acute hospitalization, have much poorer health outcomes in comparison with patients in clinical trials. For example, both Krumholz and colleagues (1997)[55] and Jaagosild and colleagues (1998)[53] have shown that in large, relatively unselected cohorts of older patients with heart failure about half of patients are readmitted within six months and one-third of patients are dead within a year. In comparison with the aforementioned studies, in the captopril arm of the ELITE study, which included older patients with a recent history of hospitalization, about 30% of patients were readmitted and 9% patients died during 48 weeks follow-up.[73]

There is little doubt that it is the type of hospitalized cohort of patients described by Lowe and colleagues (1998)[54] who consume the major share of healthcare expenditure associated with the overall management of heart failure. Moreover, any strategy designed to reduce morbidity and mortality rates while simultaneously reducing healthcare costs should therefore target patient cohorts who can be inherently characterized on the basis of being older (mean age $\geq$ 65 years), having at least one admission for acute heart failure and chronic functional impairment and having multiple, chronic disease states.

Although being older and frailer no doubt places patients with heart failure at greater risk for hospitalization and worse health outcomes thereafter, there is considerable evidence to suggest that suboptimal management of such patients may contribute significantly to their poor health outcomes. For example, part of the beneficial effects of clinical trials, as evidenced by relatively lower morbidity and mortality (despite their inherent bias towards recruiting younger, more stable and compliant patient cohorts), may be partially explained by the type of optimal treatment and intensive follow-up denied to most patients.[74] This principle is probably widely applicable – for example, it may explain in part the discrepancy between mortality data for acute myocardial infarction within and outside clinical trial participation.[75–77]

Potentially preventable factors that contribute to poor health-related quality of life, unplanned readmissions and poor survival prospects in patients with chronic congestive heart failure

The apparent inability of many individuals to gain the maximal clinical benefit from otherwise proven therapeutics is probably a multi-factorial problem.[76] This is not surprising considering the complex interaction between individuals, their treatment and the many components of the healthcare system in which they are managed. The application of a suboptimal treatment regimen (that is, one that is unlikely to have a positive impact on the health status of the patient) commonly arises from a series of problems that hinder what should be a harmonious and productive interaction between the patient and the healthcare system. The degree to which this will impact on an individual's health will undoubtedly vary, depending on the stability and severity of disease state(s) and the relative safety of the therapeutic regimen. The consequences can therefore range from lack of symptomatic control to unplanned hospitalization and even premature death. For example, it has been suggested that a significant proportion of unplanned hospital readmissions (estimates range between 9% and 54%) are preventable.[16, 25, 27, 77, 78]

Obviously, pharmacological agents such as ACE inhibitors[40, 42] and β-adreno-ceptor blockers[79, 80] have been designed to limit the physiological consequences of heart failure and have proved to be partially effective in this regard. However, even optimal combinations of pharmacological agents when closely monitored in the context of clinical trials (and their carefully selected cohorts) notably fail to eliminate all of the negative outcomes associated with heart failure. Furthermore, as noted above, most hospitalized patients fare worse than clinical trial cohorts, probably primarily because they are older, frailer and have greater co-morbidity. Although these patients would benefit most from appropriate and consistent treatment, they are, unfortunately, at greatest risk from the factors that precipitate suboptimal treatment. Furthermore, their frequent inability to tolerate even minor fluctuations in their cardiac function leaves them vulnerable to frequent and recurrent episodes of acute heart failure (in addition to acute exacerbations of concurrent disease states) and therefore frequent hospitalization. The circumstance of concomitant moderate impairment of renal function, particularly as a result of renovascular disease, in patients with chronic heart failure is of particular importance in this regard.[81] This problem is more likely to be present in elderly patients[72] and presents both an incremental hazard to the successful use of ACE inhibitors as well as a basis for increased risk of digitalis toxicity. While such patients tend to be excluded from clinical trials, their considerable prevalence in the hospitalized older population presents a therapeutic dilemma (especially in respect to balancing the risks of drug toxicity versus under-treatment) with no obvious solution.

At present the inability of current therapeutics to completely address the pathophysiological consequences of heart failure is the subject of intensive research efforts (for example, development of new pharmacological agents). However, there is little doubt that there are many preventable and often interrelated factors contributing to poorer health outcomes among patients with chronic heart failure that can be addressed through non-pharmacological means. These potentially modifiable factors can be summarized as follows:

Inadequate or inappropriate pharmacotherapy

Despite the production of clear and precise clinical guidelines for the diagnosis and management of heart failure[7–9], a large proportion of patients continue to receive suboptimal treatment.[10–12] For example, ACE inhibitors, which have undoubted cost benefits[82], are often either prescribed in subtherapeutic doses or completely (and inappropriately) omitted from a patient's treatment regimen.[10–12] Not surprisingly, patients treated by specialist cardiologists are more likely to receive appropriate treatment[32, 33, 83–86], and there is evidence, at least in some academic centres, that patients are beginning to receive more appropriate treatment.[87–88] However, most patients are treated in the community by non-specialized physicians.

Non-compliance with prescribed treatment

There is a plethora of evidence to suggest that much long-term morbidity and perhaps mortality may be related to suboptimal use and/or monitoring of prescribed pharmacotherapy. Studies examining the major determinants of poor compliance patterns among large patient populations consistently link non-adherence with the presence of chronic illness and a greater number of prescribed drugs.[89–94] Furthermore, such studies also report that close to 50% of chronically ill patients significantly deviate from prescribed pharmacotherapy.[95–98] Although it is more difficult to measure, there is little doubt that patients have similar problems adhering to fluid restrictions and salt-reduced diets.[99–100] Other frequently reported problems likely to impact on adherence include difficulty in opening medication containers[93–101], hoarding and consuming old medications[22, 91, 92], consumption of over-the-counter, non-prescribed medications likely to have a detrimental effect (for example non-steroidals[102]) and regularly altering dosages (often without informing the treating physician).[21, 92] In this respect, treating physicians frequently overestimate the extent of their patients' compliance to prescribed treatment.[21, 92] Not surprisingly, poor treatment compliance has been identified as a major precursor of readmissions among patients with chronic heart failure.[25, 56, 83]

Adverse effects of prescribed treatment

Chronically ill patients are also at increased risk of being hospitalized because of the adverse effects of their treatment, although the extent of this risk is debatable. For example, in various studies, 2–15% of hospital admissions (depending on the criteria used) among chronically ill patients have been attributed to adverse effects of prescribed medication.[22, 103] In this respect, the obvious benefits of the current pharmaco-therapeutics used in the treatment of heart failure have to be tempered by the increased risk of (among older patients especially) serious adverse effects such as deteriorating renal function secondary to ACE inhibition[104, 105], falls due to prolonged hypotension and/or severe postural hypotension secondary to vasodilator treatment[106] and digoxin toxicity secondary to the combination of overdiuresis, low fluid intake and/or impaired renal function.[107]

Inadequate knowledge of chronic heart failure and prescribed treatment

Studies have consistently shown that chronically ill patients have most difficulty in recalling the potential adverse effects and/or special instructions pertaining to their prescribed medication.[49, 54, 108, 109] This does not mean, however, that the other components of medication-related knowledge (such as understanding the purpose and intended effects of prescribed medication) are commonly known. Not surprisingly, relatively poorer health-related knowledge is frequently correlated with greater age, lower education levels and presence of a chronic illness; the typical profile of many hospitalized patients with chronic heart failure.[22]

Inadequate follow-up/suboptimal use of available health care

Both the extent of follow-up care and the ability or willingness of patients to access such care have been identified as important determinants of health outcomes among chronically ill patients.[18, 24–32] Despite the attractiveness of encouraging patients to return to their own home, rather than long-term institutional care, it is clear that such patients are at increased risk of readmission if an appropriate level of support is not provided.[110] Theoretically, providing greater follow-up care in order to increase the frequency of detecting and treating clinically unstable patients at risk of hospitalization is an attractive proposition. However, it would seem that markedly increasing patient contact with physicians who have the power to admit patients to hospital can actually increase hospitalization rates[111], most probably due to the combination of an increased likelihood of detecting usually benign fluctuations in patients' status and a lowering of the normal threshold at which patients would be hospitalized.[112]

Poor psycho-social support

Studies consistently show a close association between poorer socio-economic status and poorer health outcomes.[113–118] A major component of this risk undoubtedly relates to lack of social support, with the imposition of monetary constraints likely to limit social contacts (even via telephone) as well as buying essential items such as nutritious food and medications. Older, chronically ill patients are particularly vulnerable to these limitations and this no doubt confers an increased risk for becoming depressed and lonely, especially if they live alone.[116] Such patients also lack the support systems that would usually increase the likelihood of detecting emerging problems as well as providing both emotional and practical support in managing their chronic illness.[119]

Early clinical deterioration

Although almost all hospitalized patients with heart failure receive intensive treatment and stabilization, followed by incremental follow-up, a significant proportion (up to 20%) will rebound into hospital within a month of their discharge as a result of early clinical deterioration[54, 120], a phenomenon common to other chronic disease states.[25–28] Although the factors associated with this early 'rebound' phenomenon are poorly characterized, it is clear that older and more fragile patients with other chronic conditions that confound treatment are most at risk in this regard and that many of the factors discussed herein contribute to this phenomenon. For example, if patients with severe heart failure have been stabilized during hospitalization with a regimen requiring combined use of a loop-diuretic, spironolactone, an ACE inhibitor, a β-blocker and digoxin, there would be little doubt that they would experience marked clinical deterioration if on return home they failed to take the prescribed regimen thereafter.[107] It must also be stated, however, that increasing pressure on hospitals to discharge patients as soon as practicable is likely to result in increased risk of readmission in some borderline cases.[121] This may explain why the observed reductions in length of stay have been accompanied by an increase in the number of readmissions (data described in Chapter 3).

Summary

The dismal survival prospects associated with chronic congestive heart failure, especially among those who are older and who have symptoms refractory to what would usually be considered optimal treatment, is the reflection of a complex and debilitating syndrome that has yet to be adequately addressed. As such, older patients with heart failure who have limited treatment options face an almost inevitable cycle of clinical improvement and deterioration before dying prematurely. In the absence of pharmacological (or surgical) interventions to improve the mortality of these patients, it would seem prudent to apply strategies that maximize the time in which they are relatively stable by overcoming those factors that contribute to clinical instability. Figure 4.1 is a model of the potential determinants of the use of hospital beds (as distinct from frequency of hospitalization) by patients with chronic heart failure. It identifies potential factors impacting on healthcare costs in this regard, but does not necessarily reflect quality of life considerations for such patients.

Using the history of the variety of interventions designed to improve extent of treatment compliance among chronically ill patients as a microcosm of the complex issues that relate to the interaction between individuals, their prescribed treatment and the healthcare system in which they are managed, it is clear that multi-factorial rather than singular strategies are required to address the many complex issues that contribute to clinical instability among these patients.

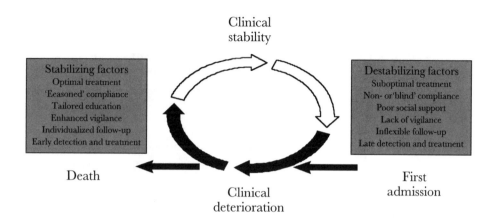

Figure 4.1: A model of the determinants of use of hospital beds among patients with chronic heart failure limited to palliative, medical therapy.

Studies of hospitalized patients with heart failure shows that once individuals develop symptomatic heart failure and survives a first hospitalization associated with acute heart failure, they are at increased risk for further hospitalization and, ultimately, premature death. For most patients the intensive treatment associated with hospitalization is linked to marked clinical improvement and subsequent discharge; although duration of stay (especially if curtailed because of budgetary pressures) may result in patients being discharged prematurely. For most patients an acute hospitalization is followed by prolonged periods of clinical stability and only infrequent (and probably unavoidable) episodes of acute deterioration, resulting, if severe enough, in an occasional unplanned readmission to hospital. Conversely, a small proportion of individuals seem to be in a continual and frequent cycle (as represented above) of clinical improvement and deterioration. Such patients are much more likely to have poorer quality of life, more severe functional impairment and recurrent (and costly) admissions to hospital. It is this type of patient who has been previously identified as the 'high-cost' user of healthcare resources, even though such patients frequently die prematurely. Inherent factors likely to determine the duration of clinical stability include (as indicated) the age of the patient, the extent of left ventricular systolic dysfunction and the extent of concomitant disease states. Similarly, interrelated external factors likely to determine clinical status include, extent of treatment compliance, medical follow-up and social support, in addition to the degree of vigilance for clinical deterioration (especially in the immediate period following hospital discharge). It is almost inevitable that patients with heart failure will die prematurely; however, the evidence suggests that there is marked variability with regard to the extent of hospital-bed use (and therefore cost of health care) in this patient population.

Figure 4.1: A model of the determinants of use of hospital beds among patients with chronic heart failure limited to palliative, medical therapy.

Furthermore, as suggested previously, the body of literature concerning heart failure and chronic illness overall suggests that those interventions that simultaneously target 'high risk' patients and the potentially modifiable factors that contribute to poorer health outcomes overall are the most likely to be cost-effective.

Chapters 5 and 6 describe a series of studies undertaken in Australia between 1995 and 2000 to determine the value of a nurse-led, multidisciplinary, home-based intervention in optimizing the post-discharge management of patients with chronic heart failure. Chapter 7 then provides a detailed discussion of the contribution of these studies to the global effort to reduce morbidity related to heart failure.

References

1. Sclarovsky S, Rechavia E, Strasberg B, et al. Unstable angina: ST segment depression with positive versus negative T wave deflections – clinical course, ECG evolution, and angiographic correlation. *Am Heart J* 1988; 116: 933–41.

2. Yusuf S, Held P, Furberg C. Update of effects of calcium antagonists in myocardial infarction or angina in light of the second Danish verapamil infarction trial (DAVIT-II) and other recent studies. *Am J Cardiol* 1991; 67: 1295–7.

3. Ronner E, Dykun Y, Van Den Brand M, et al. Platelet glycoprotein IIB/IIIA receptor antagonists: An asset for treatment of unstable coronary syndromes and coronary intervention. *Eur Heart J* 1998; 19: 1608–16.

4. Horowitz J. Role of nitrates in unstable angina pectoris. *Am Heart J* 1992; 70(suppl): 64B–70B.

5. Fox K, Antman E. Treatment options in unstable angina: A clinical update. *Eur Heart J* 1998; 19(suppl): K8–K10.

6. Maseri A, Sanna T. The role of plaque of fissures in unstable angina: Fact or fiction? *Eur Heart J* 1998; 19(suppl): K2–K4.

7. Williams J, Bristow M, Fowler M, et al. Guidelines for the evaluation and management of heart failure. Report of the American College of Cardiology/American Heart Association Task Force on Practice Guidelines (Committee on Evaluation and Management of Heart Failure). *J Am Coll Cardiol* 1995; 26: 1376–98.

8. The World Health Organization/Council on Geriatric Cardiology Task Force on Heart Failure Education. Concise guide to the management of heart failure. *Am J Geriatr Cardiol* 1996; 5: 13–30.

9. The Task Force on Heart Failure of the European Society of Cardiology. The treatment of heart failure. *Eur Heart J* 1997; 18: 736–53.

10. Ghali J, Giles T, Gonzales M, et al. Patterns of physician use of angiotensin converting enzyme inhibitors in the inpatient treatment of congestive heart failure. *J LA State Med Soc* 1997; 149: 474–84.

11. Luzier A, Forrest A, Adelman M, et al. Impact of angiotensin-converting enzyme inhibitor underdosing on rehospitalization rates in congestive heart failure. *Am J Cardiol* 1998; 82: 465–9.

12. Chronic heart failure in Australian general practice. The Cardiac Awareness Survey and Evaluation (CASE) Study. *MJA* 2001; 174: 439–44.

13. Rudd P, Ramesh J, Bryant-Kosling C, et al. Gaps in cardiovascular medication taking: The tip of the iceberg. *J Gen Intern Med* 1993; 8: 659–66.

14. Larmour I, Dolphin RG, Baxter H, et al. A prospective study of hospital admissions due to drug reactions. *Australian Journal of Hospital Pharmacy* 1991; 21: 90–5.

15. Hewitt J. Drug-related unplanned readmissions to hospital. *Australian Journal of Hospital Pharmacy* 1995; 25: 400–3.

16. Col N, Fanale JE, Kronholm P. The role of medication noncompliance and adverse drug reactions in hospitalizations of the elderly. *Arch Internal Med* 1990; 150: 841–5.

17. Dartnell JG, Anderson RP, Chohan V, et al. Hospitalisation for adverse events related to drug therapy: Incidence, avoidability and costs. *MJA* 1996; 164: 659–62.

18. Smith DM, Norton JA, McDonald CJ. Non-elective readmissions of medical patients. *J Chron Dis* 1985; 38: 213–24.

19. Hawe P, Higgins G. Can medication education improve the drug compliance of the elderly? Evaluation of an in hospital program. *Patient Educ Couns* 1990; 16: 151–60.

20. Markey BT, Igou JF. Medication discharge planning for the elderly. *Patient Educ Couns* 1987; 9: 241–9.

21. Donovan J, Blake D. Patient non-compliance: Deviance or reasoned decision-making? *Soc Sci Med* 1992; 34: 507–13.

22. Stewart S, Pearson S. Uncovering a multitude of sins: Medication management in the home post acute hospitalisation among the chronically ill. *Aust NZ J Med* 1999; 29: 220–7.

23. Weinberger M, Oddone EZ, Henderson WG. Does increased access to primary care reduce hospital readmissions? *New Engl Journal Med* 1996; 334: 1441–7.

24. Fitzgerald JF, Smith DM, Martin DK, et al. A case manager intervention to reduce readmissions. *Arch Intern Med* 1994; 154: 1721–9.

25. Graham H, Livesley B. Can readmissions to a geriatric medical unit be prevented? *Lancet* 1983; i: 404–6.

26. Ashton CM, Kuykendall DH, Johnson ML, et al. The association between quality of inpatient care and early readmission. *Ann Intern Med* 1995; 122: 415–21.

27. Ashton CM, Wray NP, Dunn KJ, et al. Predicting readmission in veterans with chronic disease. *Med Care* 1986; 25: 1184–9.

28. Evans RL, Hendricks RD, Lawrence KV, et al. Identifying factors associated with health care use: A hospital-based screening index. *Soc Scient Med* 1988; 27: 947–54.

29. Evans RL, Hendricks RD. Evaluating hospital discharge planning: A randomized clinical trial. *Med Care* 1993; 31: 358–70.

30. Naylor M, Brooten D, Jones R, et al. Comprehensive discharge planning for the hospitalized elderly. *Ann Intern Med* 1994; 120: 999–1006.

31. Smith DM, Weinberger M, Katz BP, et al. Post discharge care and readmissions. *Med Care* 1988; 26: 699–708.

32. Kelly J, McDowell H, Crawford V, et al. Readmissions to a geriatric medical unit: Is prevention possible? *Aging* 1992; 4: 61–7.

33. Stewart S, Pearson S, Luke CG, et al. Effects of a home-based intervention on unplanned readmissions and out-of-hospital deaths. *J Am Geriatr Soc* 1998; 46: 174–80.

34. Krum H. Reducing the burden of chronic heart failure (editorial). *MJA* 1997; 167: 61–2.

35. Petrie M, Berry C, Stewart S, et al. Failing ageing hearts. *Eur Heart J* 2001: 22: 1978–90.

36. McMurray JJV, Stewart S. Epidemiology, aetiology and prognosis of heart failure. *Heart* 2000; 83: 596–602.

37. Mark DB. Economics of treating heart failure. *Am J Cardiol* 1997; 80(8B): 33H–38H.

38. O'Connor C, Gattis W, Swedburg K. Current and novel pharmacological approaches in advanced heart failure. *Am Heart J* 1998; 135(suppl): S249–263.

39. McDonagh TA, Morrison CE, Lawrence A, et al. Symptomatic and asymptomatic left-ventricular systolic dysfunction in an urban population. *Lancet* 1997; 350: 829–33.

40. McClure S, Caruana L, Davie J, et al. Heart failure diagnosis by natriuretic peptide measurement. Does it work in clinical practice? *Eur Heart J* 1998; 19(suppl): 249.

41. McClure S, Caruana L, Davie J, et al. Heart failure diagnosis by natriuretic peptide measurement. Does it work in clinical practice? *Eur Heart J* 1998; 19(Suppl): 249.

42. The SOLVD Investigators. Effect of enalapril on mortality and the development of heart failure in asymptomatic patients with reduced left ventricular ejection fractions. *N Engl J Med* 1992; 327: 685–91.

43. Andersson B, Waagstein F. Spectrum and outcome of congestive heart failure in a hospitalized population. *Am Heart J* 1993; 126: 632–40.

44. Franciosa JA, Wilen M, Ziesche S, et al. Survival in men with severe chronic left ventricular failure due to either coronary heart disease or idiopathic dilated cardiomyopathy. *Am J Cardiol* 1983; 51: 831–6.

45. Stevenson W, Middlekauff H, Stevenson L, et al. Significance of aborted cardiac arrests and sustained ventricular tachycardia in patients referred for treatment of advanced heart failure. *Am Heart J* 1992; 124: 123–30.

46. Kelly T, Cremo R, Nielsen C, et al. Predictions of outcome in late-stage cardiomyopathy. *Am Heart J* 1990; 119: 1111–21.

47. Glover DR, Littler WL. Factors influencing survival and mode of death in severe chronic ischaemic cardiac failure. *Br Heart J* 1987; 57: 125–32.

48. Willenheimer R, Erhardt L, Cline C, et al. Prognostic significance of changes in left ventricular systolic function in elderly patients with congestive heart failure. *Coron Artery Dis* 1997; 8: 711–17.

49. Blyth F, Lazarus R, Ross D, et al. Burden and outcomes of hospitalisation for congestive heart failure. *MJA* 1997; 167: 67–70.

50. Chin MH, Goldman L. Correlates of major complications or death in patients admitted to the hospital with congestive heart failure. *Arch Intern Med* 1996; 156: 1814–20.

51. Ni H, Nauman D, Hershberger R. Managed care and outcomes of hospitalization among elderly patients with congestive heart failure. *Arch Intern Med* 1998; 158: 1231–6.

52. Setaro JF, Soufer R, Remetz MS, et al. Long-term outcome in patients with congestive heart failure and intact systolic left ventricular performance. *Am J Cardiol* 1992; 69: 1212–16.

53. Jaagosild P, Dawson N, Thomas C, et al. Outcomes of acute exacerbation of severe congestive heart failure. *Arch Intern Med* 1998; 158: 1081–9.

54. Lowe J, Candlish P, Henry D, et al. Management and outcomes of congestive heart failure: A prospective study of hospitalised patients. *MJA* 1998; 168: 115–18.

55. Krumholz HM, Parent EM, Tu N, et al. Readmission after hospitalization for congestive heart failure among medicare beneficiaries. *Arch Intern Med* 1997; 157: 99–104.

56. Vinson JM, Rich MW, Sperry JC, et al. Early readmission of elderly patients with congestive heart failure. *J Am Geriatr Soc* 1990; 38: 1290–5.

57. Wolinsky F, Smith D, Stump T, et al. The sequelae of hospitalization for congestive heart failure among older adults. *J Am Geriatr Soc* 1997; 45: 558–63.

58. Sugrue D, Rodeheffer R, Codd M, et al. The clinical course of idiopathic dilated cardiomyopathy. A population-based study. *Ann Intern Med* 1992; 117: 117–23.

59. Bart B, Shaw L, McCants C, et al. Clinical determinants of mortality in patients with angiographically diagnosed ischemic or nonischemic cardiomyopathy. *J Am Coll Cardiol* 1997; 30: 1002–8.

60. Gurwitz J, Col N, Avorn J. The exclusion of the elderly and women from clinical trials in acute myocardial infarction. *JAMA* 1992; 268: 1417–22.

61. Cohen-Solal A, Delahaye F, Desnos M, et al. Who are the patients hospitalised for heart failure in France today? (Abstract). *Eur Heart J* 1998; 19(suppl): 248.

62. Pitt B, Chang P, Timmermans P. Angiotensin II receptor antagonists in heart failure: Rationale and design of the Evaluation of Losartan in the Elderly (ELITE) trial. *Cardiovasc Drug Ther* 1995; 9: 693–700.

63. Hampton J, van Veldhuisen D, Kleber F, et al. Randomised study of ibopamine on survival in patients with advanced severe heart failure (Prime II). *Lancet* 1997; 349: 971–7.

64. Aronow W, Ahn C, Kronzon I. Normal left ventricular ejection fraction in older persons with congestive heart failure. *Chest* 1998; 113: 867–9.

65. Doughty RN, Wright SP, Walsh HJ, et al. Randomised, controlled trial of integrated heart failure management: The Auckland Heart Failure Management Study. *Eur Heart J* 2002; 23: 139–46.

66. Crijns HJ, Van den Berg MP, Van Gelder IC, et al. Management of atrial fibrillation in the setting of heart failure. *Eur Heart J* 1997; 18: C45–9.

67. Van den Berg MP, Tuinenburg AE, Crijns HJ, et al. Heart failure and atrial fibrillation: Current concepts and controversies. *Heart* 1997; 77: 309–13.

68. Goldberger MJ, Peled HB, Stroh JA, et al. Prognostic factors in acute pulmonary edema. *Arch Intern Med* 1986; 146: 489–93.

69. Cowburn P, Cleland J, Coats A, et al. Risk stratification in chronic heart failure. *Eur Heart J* 1998; 19: 696-710.

70. Maggioni A, De Santis F, Fabbri G, et al. Predictors of hospital admission in patients with congestive heart failure: Data from Italian network on congestive heart failure (Abstract). *Eur Heart J* 1998; 19(suppl): 249.

71. Walsh J, Charlesworth A, Andrews A, et al. Relation of daily activity levels in patients with chronic heart failure to long-term prognosis. *Am J Cardiol* 1997; 79: 1364–9.

72. Brown A, Cleland J. Influence of concomitant disease on patterns of hospitalization in patients with heart failure discharged from Scottish hospitals in 1995. *Eur Heart J* 1998; 19: 1063–9.

73. Pitt B, Poole-Wilson PA, Segal R, et al, on behalf of the ELITE-II Investigators. Effect of losartan compared with captopril on mortality in patients with symptomatic heart failure: Randomised trial – the Losartan Heart Failure Survival Study Elite-II. *Lancet* 2000; 355: 1582–7.

74. Tu J, Chris L, Pashos C, et al. Use of cardiac procedures and outcomes in elderly patients with myocardial infarction in the United States and Canada. *N Engl J Med* 1997; 336: 1500–5.

75. Ellerbeck E, Jencks S, Radford M, et al. Quality of care for Medicare patients with acute myocardial infarction. *JAMA* 1995; 273: 1509–14.

76. Strömberg A, Broström A, Dahlström B, et al. Patient compliance with heart failure treatment. *Eur Heart J* 1998; 19(suppl): 230.

77. Lakshmanan MC, Hershey CO, Breslau D. Hospital admissions caused by iatrogenic disease. *Arch Intern Med* 1986; 146: 1931–4.

78. Clarke A. Are readmissions avoidable? *BMJ* 1990; 301: 1136–8.

79. CIBIS II Investigators. The Cardiac Insufficiency Bisoprolol Study II (CIBIS II): A randomised trial. *Lancet* 1999; 353: 9–13.

80. Packer M, Coats AJS, Fowler MB, et al., for the Carvedilol Prospective Randomized Cumulative Survival (COPERNICUS) Study Group. *N Engl J Med* 2001; 344: 1651–8.

81. MacDowall P, Kaira P, O'Donoghue D, et al. Risk of morbidity from renovascular disease in elderly patients with congestive cardiac failure. *Lancet* 1998; 352: 13–16.

82. McMurray J, Davie A. The pharmacoeconomics of ACE inhibitors in chronic heart failure. *PharmacoEconomics* 1996; 9: 188–97.

83. Rich M, Brooks K, Luther P. Temporal trends in pharmacotherapy for congestive heart failure at an academic medical centre: 1990–1995. *Am Heart J* 1998; 135: 367–72.

84. Horowitz JD, Stewart S. Heart failure in the elderly – the epidemic we had to have (Editorial). *MJA 2001*; 174: 432–3.

85. Stafford RS, Saglam D, Blumenthal D. National patterns of angiotensin-converting enzyme inhibitor use in congestive heart failure. *Arch Intern Med* 1997; 157: 2460–4.

86. Pearson TA, Peters TD. The treatment gap in coronary artery disease and heart failure: Community standards and the post-discharge patient. *Am J Cardiol* 1997; 80(suppl): 45H–52H.

87. McLaughlin T, Soumerai S, Willison D, et al. Adherence to national guidelines for drug treatment of suspected acute myocardial infarction: Evidence for undertreatment in women and the elderly. *Arch Intern Med* 1996; 156: 799–805.

88. McDermott M, Lee P, Mehta S, et al. Patterns of angiotensin-converting enzyme inhibitor prescriptions, educational interventions, and outcomes among hospitalized patients with heart failure. *Clin Cardiol* 1998; 21: 261–8.

89. Lowe CJ, Raynor DK, Courtney EA, et al. Effects of self medication programme on knowledge of drugs and compliance with treatment in elderly patients. *BMJ* 1995; 310: 1229–31.

90. Wright E. Non-compliance – or how many aunts has Matilda? *Lancet* 1993; 342: 909–13.

91. Stewart S, Davey M, Desanctis M, et al. Home medication management: A study of patient post-hospitalisation. *Australian Pharmacist* 1995; 14: 472–6.

92. Parkin D, Henney C, Quirk J, et al. Deviation from prescribed drug treatment after discharge from hospital. *BMJ* 1976; 2: 686–8.

93. Nikolaus T, Kruse W, Bach M, et al. Elderly patients' problems with medication. An in-hospital and follow-up study. *Euro J Clin Pharmacol* 1996; 49: 255–9.

94. Graveley EA, Oseasohn CS. Multiple drug regimens: Medication compliance among veterans 65 years and older. *Research in Nursing and Health* 1991; 14: 51–8.

95. Eraker SA, Kirscht JP, Becker MH. Understanding and improving patient compliance. *Ann Intern Med* 1984; 100: 258–68.

96. Spagnoli A, Ostino G, Borga AD, et al. Drug compliance and unreported drugs in the elderly. *J Am Geriatr Soc* 1989; 37: 619–24.

97. Sackett D, Haynes R, Gibson E, et al. Randomised clinical trial of strategies for medication compliance in primary hypertension. *Lancet* 1975; 1: 1265–8.

98. Haynes B, McKibbon K, Kanai R. Systematic review of randomised trials of interventions to assist patients to follow prescriptions for medications. *Lancet* 1996; 348: 383–6.

99. West J, Miller N, Parker K, et al. A comprehensive management system for heart failure improves clinical outcomes and reduces medical resource utilization. *Am J Cardiol* 1997; 79: 58–63.

100. Happ M, Naylor M, Roe-Prior P. Factors contributing to rehospitalization of elderly patients with heart failure. *J Cardiovasc Nurs* 1997; 11: 75–84.

101. Blenkiron P. The elderly and their medication: Understanding and compliance in a family practice. *Postgrad Med J* 1996; 72: 671–6.

102. Heerdink E, Leufkens H, Herings R, et al. NSAIDs associated with increased risk of congestive heart failure in elderly patients taking diuretics. *Arch Intern Med* 1998; 158: 1108–12.

103. Hallas J, Harvald B, Gram L, et al. Drug related hospital admissions: The role of definitions and intensity of data collection, and the possibility of prevention. *J Intern Med* 1990;

228: 83–90.

104. Dzau V. Vascular and renal prostaglandins as counter-regulatory systems in heart failure. *Eur Heart J* 1988; 9(suppl): H15–H19.

105. Pearson T, Pittman D, Longley J, et al. Factors associated with preventable adverse drug reactions. *Am J Hosp Pharm* 1994; 51: 2268–72.

106. Tinetti M, Baker D, McAvay G, et al. A multifactorial intervention to reduce the risk of falling among elderly people living in the community. *N Engl J Med* 1994; 331: 821–7.

107. Kirkwood F, Gheorghiade M, Uretsky B, et al. Patients with mild heart failure worsen during withdrawal from digoxin therapy. *J Am Coll Cardiol* 1997; 30: 42–8.

108. Furlong S. Do programmes of medicine self-administration enhance patient knowledge, compliance and satisfaction? *J Adv Nurs* 1996; 23: 1254–62.

109. Veggeland T, Fagerheim KU, Ritland T, et al. Do patients know enough about their medication? A questionnaire among cardiac patients discharged from 5 Norwegian hospitals. *Tidsskrift for Den Norske Laegeforening* 1993; 113: 3013–16.

110. Camberg L, Smith N, Beaudet M, et al. Discharge destination and repeat hospitalizations. *Med Care* 1997; 35: 756–67.

111. Weinberger M, Oddone EZ, Henderson WG. Does increased access to primary care reduce hospital readmissions? *New Engl Journal Med* 1996; 334: 1441–7.

112. Mold JW, Stein HF. The cascade effect in the clinical care of patients. *New Engl J Med* 1986: 512–14.

113. Bartley M, Owen C. Relation between socio-economic status, employment, and health during economic change, 1973–93. *BMJ* 1996; 313: 445–9.

114. Epstein A, Stern R, Weissman J. Do the poor cost more? A multihospital study of patients' socioeconomic status and use of hospital resources. *N Engl J Med* 1990; 322: 1122–8.

115. Glover J, Sharnd M, Foster C, et al. A social health atlas of South Australia (2nd edition). Adelaide: Policy and Budget Division, South Australian Health Commission, 1996.

116. Penninx B, van Tilburg T, Kriegsman D, et al. Effects of social support and personal coping resources on mortality in older age: The Longitudinal Aging Study Amsterdam. *Am J Epidemiol* 1997; 146: 510–19.

117. MacIntyre K, Stewart S, Capewell S, et al. Heart of inequality – the relationship between socio-economic deprivation and death from a first acute myocardial infarction: A population-based analysis. *BMJ* 2001; 322: 1152–3.

118. Morrisson C, Woodward M, Leslie W, et al. Effect of socio-economic group on the incidence of, management of and survival after myocardial infarction and coronary death; analysis of community coronary event register. *BMJ* 1997; 314: 541–6.

119. Lledo R, Martin E, Jimenz C, et al. Characteristics of elderly inpatients at high risk of needing supportive social and health care services. *Eur J Epidemiol* 1997; 13: 903–7.

120. Rich MW, Vinson JM, Sperry JC, et al. Prevention of readmission in elderly patients with congestive heart failure: Results of a prospective, randomized pilot study. *J Gen Intern Med* 1993; 8: 585–90.

121. Gooding J, Jette AM. Hospital readmissions among the elderly. *J Am Geriatr Soc* 1985; 33: 595–601.

CHAPTER 5

Preliminary studies of home-based intervention

Introduction

As discussed in the previous chapters, like other chronically ill patients, older and frailer patients with heart failure who require acute hospitalization are at greater risk for hospital readmission and premature death. So, there is a clear need to target patients at higher risk for recurrent hospital use with adjunctive, non-pharmacological interventions that address many of the preventable precursors to hospital admission/readmission. Those interventions that involve both home visits and a multidisciplinary approach coordinated by a specialist nurse seem to offer the greatest likelihood of reducing hospital use among 'high risk' patients.

It is in this context that the following studies were performed to examine the potential benefits of a relatively cheap, multidisciplinary, home-based intervention in limiting hospital readmission and prolonging survival in chronically ill patients.[1–3]

Methods

Study hypothesis

This study tested the following *null hypothesis*: There will be no difference in the frequency of the primary end-point of unplanned readmission plus out-of-hospital death during six-month follow-up among chronically ill cardiac and non-cardiac patients discharged to home following acute hospitalization on the basis of exposure/non-exposure to a post-discharge, multidisciplinary, home-based intervention (HBI) incremental to usual care.

Patient population

The study was conducted at the Queen Elizabeth Hospital, a 440-bed hospital servicing the northwestern region of Adelaide, South Australia, an area with a disproportionate number of elderly and socially disadvantaged people. The link between predominantly socially disadvantaged, elderly populations and poorer health outcomes in Australia[4] is reflected in the high levels of chronic illness and higher admission rates per capita for the region.[5]

Eligibility criteria

All patients admitted to medical and surgical units at the hospital were eligible to participate in the study if they were to be discharged to their own home and prescribed a medication regimen for at least one chronic illness.

Exclusion criteria

Patients were excluded, however, if they were: a) diagnosed with a terminal malignancy requiring palliative care; b) scheduled for an elective admission within the study period of six months; or c) residing at a home address that was outside the hospital's usual catchment area.

Prior to patient recruitment, the hospital's Ethics of Human Research Committee approved the study. During a 12-month period, 4100 medical and surgical patients were screened, of whom 22% (n = 906) were considered eligible for the study. Of these, 762 (84%) agreed to participate. The baseline characteristics of participating patients were similar to those of the subset of eligible patients who refused to participate in the study. The predominant reasons for patient refusal included anticipated intrusiveness of a home visit and/or a belief that the intervention would be of little benefit.

Informed consent was obtained before discharge from hospital and participating patients were randomized to either usual care (UC) or HBI. Patients were randomized via a telephone call to an investigator blinded to the patient's demographic and clinical profile but aware of their medical or surgical admission status. Using a computer-generated, stratified randomization program, patients were allocated to either HBI or UC according to their medical or surgical admission status, to correct for potential imbalance between groups.

Immediately after randomization an initial interview was conducted with all patients to document their baseline characteristics, including extent of concurrent illness using the Charlson Index of Co-morbidity.[6] During this initial assessment, the presence or absence of the following, previously reported risk factors for unplanned hospitalization was identified: age $\geq$ 60 years, prescription of $\geq$ two medications, unplanned admission within preceding six months, living alone and/or possessing limited English language skills.[7–12] Patients with multiple risk factors were prospectively designated as 'high risk' for unplanned readmission during study follow-up; other patients were designated as 'low risk'.

Patient management

Pre-discharge counselling

The intensity of study intervention in the HBI group was dependent on the initial assessment of risk. As such, all patients and caregivers in the HBI group (n = 381) were counselled before discharge by the study nurse and/or hospital pharmacist in relation to compliance with prescribed medication and early detection/reporting of clinical deterioration. The post-hospitalization intervention, however, was confined to those HBI patients with multiple risk factors and therefore designated as 'high risk' (n = 314). This subset of patients represented 82% of HBI patients.

Home-based assessment and intervention

One week after discharge high-risk HBI patients were subject to a single home visit by the study nurse and pharmacist (the same two people performed all of the home visits during the study). The prospectively designated objectives of this home visit were principally four-fold:

1. To optimize home-medication management.
2. To detect problems that would have otherwise remained undetected.
3. To increase patient and/or carer vigilance for clinical deterioration and therefore an impending crisis if not treated promptly.
4. To improve liaison with community-based services thereafter on the basis of a more accurate assessment of the patient's needs in their own home.

For research purposes only (because a small subset of 'high-risk' UC patients were designated to receive an abbreviated home visit), during the initial stage of this home visit the study nurse performed a *blinded* review of the patient's management of their medication regimen. This involved assessment of the following:

Medication compliance

A pill count of the seven-day supply of medications given to the patient at hospital discharge was done to compare the patient's expected versus actual consumption of oral tablets. It is important to note that patients were unaware before the home visit that a pill count would be done. Patients were considered to be compliant if they had consumed 85–115% of the prescribed number of tablets.

Medication-related knowledge

Using a structured questionnaire, patients (and/or appropriate carers) were asked to name the following knowledge components relating to their prescribed regimen in the following order: primary purpose, dosage, frequency, special instructions and potential adverse effects for each medication. Individual responses relating to the first four components were dichotomously rated as correct or incorrect by the study pharmacist who, before each home visit, had prospectively designated adequate responses for each prescribed medication. Scores were then averaged for each component (for example, patients scored 75% for correctly identifying the purpose of six out of eight prescribed drugs). Responses to the potential adverse effects were scored, unlike the other components, on a continuum from excellent (100% for identifying all major adverse effects relevant to each medication), through very good (75%), fair (50%), poor (25%) to very poor (0% – unable to identify any adverse effects). Once a criterion had been developed for a particular medication (for example, captopril), it was retained for all subsequent home visits. On the basis of all individual component scores given by the patient (an average of 30 a patient), an overall, average knowledge score of 0–100% was calculated. On this basis, a patient who scored ≥ 75% in response to the questionnaire was considered to have 'adequate' medication-related knowledge.

General pattern of medication management

Using a structured 18-item general-purpose questionnaire developed during the pilot study[7], patients were also asked a series of questions concerning any potential difficulties they experienced in relation to obtaining, consuming and monitoring their medication regimen.

Patients whose compliance deviated by ≥ 15% from prescribed dosage at discharge or whose medication knowledge was considered inadequate (< 75% composite knowledge score of dosage, intended effect, potential side effects and special instructions) were then offered a combination of the following:

1. Immediate remedial counselling by the nurse and pharmacist.
2. Introduction of a compliance device and/or daily routine to assist compliance with the prescribed regimen.
3. Incremental monitoring of their clinical status via their family members and friends, or, if necessary, by their general practitioner, community nurse or community pharmacist.
4. Provision of a medication information/reminder card that could be updated by the patient's general practitioner or pharmacist.
5. Referral to a community pharmacist for regular review of potential problems thereafter (for example, during each visit to the pharmacy to collect prescribed medication).

Following the intervention by the pharmacist, the study nurse assessed the patient in order to detect any clinical deterioration since discharge. This involved both a physical assessment and a review of relevant symptoms since hospital discharge (for example, degree of exercise intolerance among patients with congestive heart failure). Those needing medical review were immediately referred to their community-based physician for a more detailed and definitive assessment. The study nurse also reviewed the patients' psychosocial status in order to determine the need (if any) for additional community-based support. In this respect, the patients' ability to maintain and monitor their health, especially in the absence of proximal caregivers, was of particular concern. Patients requiring additional support were referred to an appropriate community-based health professional/ organization.

After the home visit, all of the patients' general practitioners were contacted by the study nurse to inform them of the HBI and to discuss the need for further remedial action and/or more intensive follow-up. Importantly, the extent of HBI was not increased in any patients in the HBI group who needed to be readmitted during the study.

Usual post-discharge care

Patients in the UC group (n = 381) were not limited in the frequency and duration of pre-existing levels of health care. In this respect, all patients were subject to the hospital's usual process of discharge planning and arrangement of post-hospitalization care; depending on patients' individual needs. As such, all UC patients had appointments to be reviewed by their primary care physician and/or hospital physician (in the hospital's outpatient department) within two weeks of discharge. Furthermore, no restriction was imposed on the extent of home-based care (for example, regular community nurse visits). As mentioned above, in order to assess for potential confounding differences in the pattern of post-discharge medication management, and using the same methodology as was used for the initial blinded assessment of HBI patients, 84 high-risk UC patients received an abbreviated home visit at one week to determine their levels of compliance and medication knowledge.

Study end-points

Primary end-point

The prospectively designated primary end-point for this study was the number of unplanned readmissions within six months of the index admission *plus* out-of-hospital deaths (weighted as the equivalent of one 'unplanned readmission'). This combined mortality and readmission end-point was chosen, as in other previously reported studies[13], to adjust partially for the potential reduction in readmissions if patients died outside of the hospital.

Secondary end-points

Prospectively defined secondary end-points for the study were the number of unplanned readmissions, total days of hospital readmission (as a result of elective plus unplanned readmissions), number of emergency service attendances, out-of-hospital mortality, overall mortality and total cost of hospital-based health care.

Data collection

Hospital use and survival data

All inpatient and outpatient activity was monitored through the hospital's computerized medical records system. Records of the time and location of all deaths occurring in South Australia (available through the South Australian Birth, Deaths and Marriages Registry) were used to compile mortality data.

Healthcare costs

Cost of hospital admissions and outpatient appointments were calculated using the hospital's inpatient and outpatient costing system. Costs associated with the study intervention were calculated for the entire HBI group. Calculation of these costs included:

1. Salary for the study nurse and pharmacist as determined by detailed diary entries.
2. Use of other professional services (for example, interpreting)
3. Infrastructure requirements (for example, personal communications and transport)
4. Additional consultation with a community pharmacist.

A detailed costing of community-based healthcare costs (other than study intervention) was also performed in 150 randomly selected patients. Calculation of these costs included the following components:

1. Consultation with general practitioners (according to standard Medicare fees).
2. Prescribed pharmacotherapy (according to standard pharmaceutical costs).
3. Home visits by healthcare professionals.

Health-related quality of life

For comparative purposes, randomly selected HBI and UC patients were interviewed by telephone, by a blinded investigator, to determine the quality of life of surviving patients at one and three months using the Australian version of the SF-36 health-related quality of life questionnaire.[14] The SF-36 is a brief general health status measure, whose validity and reliability in discriminating between patient populations has been confirmed in the United States[15] and Australia.[14] This questionnaire measures the following eight dimensions of health:

1. Limitations in physical activities because of health problems.
2. Limitations in usual role activities because of physical health problems.
3. Bodily pain.
4. General health perception.
5. Vitality.
6. Limitations in social activities because of physical or emotional problems.
7. Limitations in usual role activities because of emotional problems.
8. Mental health.

In addition, these scales can be combined to represent two summary measures of physical and mental health. Responses to the questions on each scale are summed to provide scores between 0 and 100, with higher scores indicative of better health.[16] In order to maximize the response rate and consistency of measurements for the 180 patients randomly assigned to measurement of health-related quality of life (HRQL) at one month after acute hospitalization, all responses to the SF-36 were elicited by the same investigator during a telephone interview; this method of administering the SF-36 has been shown to be as reliable and as valid as a face-to-face interview.[17]

Statistical analysis

Pilot data suggested that the rate of unplanned readmission plus out-of-hospital death would be about 0.5 events per patient during six-month follow-up. We therefore calculated that 380 patients in each group would be required to detect a 10% variation in this composite end-point with a = 0.05 and b = 0.2. Comparison of baseline and end-point data involved using the following:

1. Chi-square analysis (with calculation of odds ratio – OR and 95% confidence intervals) for discrete variables.
2. Student's t test for normally distributed continuous variables.
3. Mann-Whitney U test for non-normally distributed variables without a large proportion of tied observations.
4. Z-test of two independent counts for variables with a large proportion of tied observations.
5. Log-rank test for analysis of the mortality data (Kaplan-Meier curve) and time to first unplanned readmission. All analyses were performed on an *intention-to-treat* basis and included data from the entire cohort (n = 782) for all major end-points.

Comparison of the eight health dimension scores generated by the SF-36 was made with the Bonferonni *t* test for multiple comparisons (adjusted a of 0.05/8 = 0.006).

To determine independent correlates of the clinical outcomes measured as part of the study (including the two composites of the primary end-point), multiple logistical regression (with entry of univariate variables at an α level of 0.2 and stepwise rejection of variables at the conventional a level of 0.05) was performed. Figure 5.1 represents a schema of the study methodology, summarizing the important points discussed in the methods section.

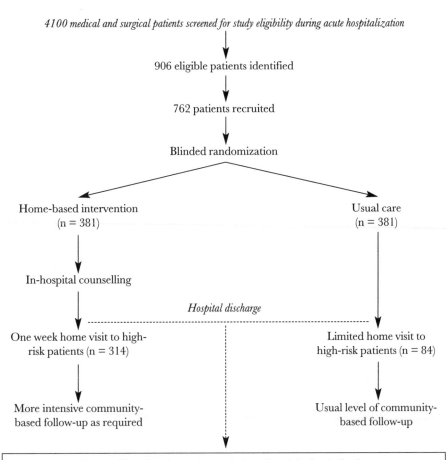

4100 medical and surgical patients screened for study eligibility during acute hospitalization

906 eligible patients identified

762 patients recruited

Blinded randomization

Home-based intervention
(n = 381)

Usual care
(n = 381)

In-hospital counselling

Hospital discharge

One week home visit to high-risk patients (n = 314)

Limited home visit to high-risk patients (n = 84)

More intensive community-based follow-up as required

Usual level of community-based follow-up

Patients followed for six months post discharge from index hospitalization

Primary end-point = frequency of unplanned readmissions plus out-of-hospital deaths

Secondary end-points = total hospital stay, emergency service contacts, survival and hospital-based costs in all patients, health-related quality of life and community-based costs among randomly selected patients

Figure 5.1: Study schema: patient recruitment, randomization and follow-up.

Results

Baseline characteristics

Table 5.1 summarizes the clinical and demographic features of study patients according to treatment group. Analysis of baseline data, including extent of comorbidity, suggested that the groups were well matched as there were no statistical differences in any of the parameters examined. Most people in the study cohort were elderly, of low socio-economic status and were frequently being treated for multiple chronic illnesses with ≥ two prescribed medications. Despite initial informed consent, 56 (18%) high-risk HBI patients did not receive a home visit (usually because of withdrawal of consent); this subsequent refusal rate is consistent with studies examining similar interventions.

Table 5.1: Clinical and demographic characteristics of 782 chronically ill patients randomized to home-based intervention or usual care (all numbers in parentheses are %).

	Home-based intervention (n = 381)	Usual care (n = 381)
Demographic profile		
Age in years (mean ± SD)	66.0 ± 15.7	65.3 ± 15.8
Male : Female	193 : 188	191 : 190
Socio-economic status		
Employed (full- or part-time)	42 (11)	50 (13)
Recipient of government pension	305 (80)	306 (80)
Married/de facto	204 (54)	207 (54)
Live alone	132 (35)	124 (33)
Non-English speaking	43 (11)	49 (13)
Formal education ≤ 8 years in total	263 (69)	263 (69)
Clinical profile		
Pre-existing treatment for chronic condition	321 (84)	323 (84)
Charlson Co-morbidity Index (mean ± SD)	1.3 ± 0.7	1.3 ± 0.6
Number of patients with an unplanned admission 6 months prior to follow-up	273 (72)	283 (74)
Number of patients with multiple unplanned admissions 6 months prior to follow-up	65 (17)	67 (17)
Days of unplanned hospitalization 6 months prior to follow-up (mean ± sd)	2674 (7.0 ± 8.1)	2694 (7.1 ± 9.1)
Type of index admission		
Unplanned for a pre-existing chronic illness	107 (28)	120 (32)
Unplanned for a new onset, acute illness	162 (43)	152 (40)
Elective	112 (29)	109 (28)

Table 5.1: (contd).

	Home-based intervention (n = 381)	Usual care (n = 381)
Category of primary diagnosis		
Cardiac disease	99 (26)	113 (30)
Respiratory disease	52 (14)	41 (11)
Orthopaedic condition	67 (18)	65 (17)
Vascular disease	57 (14)	61 (16)
Other	106 (28)	101 (27)
Discharge medications		
Number of prescribed medications (mean ± SD)	4.8 ± 2.8	4.7 ± 2.5
Assessed risk for an unplanned readmission		
within 6 months of follow-up		
High risk (≥ two risk factors)	314 (82)	318 (84)
Low risk	67 (18)	63 (16)

There were no statistically significant differences between groups on the basis of clinical and demographic characteristics measured at baseline.

Nature of multidisciplinary, home-based intervention

Table 5.2 is a summary of the medications prescribed to the 314 'high-risk' patients (258 HBI and 84 UC patients) who received a home visit and were subject to the initial, blinded assessment of medication management by the study pharmacist. Most patients were prescribed chronic pharmacotherapy for either a chronic cardiovascular (the most common being ischaemic heart disease and/or congestive heart failure) or respiratory condition (most commonly chronic airways limitation). During 156/342 of these home visits the study pharmacist was unable to identify all the original medications dispensed at hospital discharge. The principal reason for the non-identification of hospital-derived medication was the combined presence of hospital-derived medication, pre-existing medications and those recently prescribed by the patient's general practitioner, usually since hospital discharge. Consequently, a complete and 'accurate' pill count was possible for 186 of the cohort (54%). On the basis of these pill counts, 86 patients (46%) were found to be malcompliant with their prescribed medication regimen. Of the remaining patients who were not subject to a 'reliable' pill count, 35 (22%) reported that they had completely omitted taking one or more of their prescribed medications. There were no differences between groups as regards extent of compliance.

Only 14 patients achieved a perfect score for each component of medication-related knowledge relating to the primary purpose, frequency, dosage,

Table 5.2: Most commonly prescribed medications among the cohort of 'high-risk' study patients subject to a home visit at one week post discharge

Pharmacotherapy	n = 342 (%)
Anti-platelet/anti-coagulant	181 (53)
Bronchodilator(s)	124 (36)
Diuretic(s)	123 (36)
Steroidal/non-steroidal anti-inflammatory	109 (32)
Anti-arrhythmic(s)	106 (31)
Prophylactic nitrate	92 (27)
ACE inhibitor	88 (26)
H_2 antagonist	87 (26)

potential adverse effects and special instructions for their medication regimen; most other patients achieved scores of $\leq 75\%$ and were therefore considered to have 'inadequate' knowledge. Table 5.3 summarizes the results of the medication questionnaire and presents both individual component scores and composite scores. In this respect, patients were best able to recall the general purpose, dosage and frequency of their medication regimen while demonstrating much poorer knowledge concerning potential adverse effects and/or special instructions.

Table 5.3: Extent of medication-related knowledge assessed at one week post discharge

Component of medication-related knowledge (%)	n = 342 (%)
Primary purpose	87.6 ± (23.0)
Dosage	94.7 ± (15.3)
Frequency	94.3 ± (16.0)
Special instructions	19.7 ± (18.9)
Potential adverse effects	8.7 ± (13.8)
Composite score	61.0 ± (10.9)

On the basis of multivariate analysis, greater age, less formal education and an index hospitalization primarily caused by an acute exacerbation of a preexisting chronic illness were independently correlated with a relatively lower composite score for medication-related knowledge: relatively 'higher' and 'lower' knowledge scores were determined on the basis of their relationship to the mean composite score of 63% for the entire cohort. In this respect, inhospital counselling was not associated with incremental knowledge scores. Similarly, the only independent correlate of malcompliance (using data from the 186 'reliable' pill counts) was greater number of prescribed medications. These data are summarized in Table 5.4.

Table 5.4: Correlates of degree of compliance and extent of knowledge in relation to the post-discharge medication regimen

	Knowledge score (n = 342)		p value		
	High (n = 156)	Low n = 186	Univariate analysis	Multivariate analysis	Adjusted OR (95% CI)
Age (years)	67.4 ± 12.1	72.3 ± 10.4	< 0.001	< 0.001	2.2* (1.4, 3.7)
Acute exacerbation of a chronic illness	138 (74%)	179 (96%)	0.03	0.044	2.7 (1.1, 7.1)
Primary school education only	48 (31%)	79 (43%)	< 0.01	< 0.004	1.9 (1.2, 3.0)

	Compliance (n = 186)		p value		
	Compliant (n = 100)	Malcompliant (n = 86)	Univariate analysis	Multivariate analysis	Adjusted OR (95% CI)
Mean number of discharge medications	5.1 ± 2.3	5.8 ± 2.1	0.01	< 0.002	2.6** (1.4–5.2)

*Adjusted odds ratio for ≥ 75 years. ** Adjusted odds ratio for ≥ 5 medications.

Responses to the general medication questionnaire revealed a number of other issues likely to positively or negatively impact on longer-term compliance and/or efficacy of the medication regimen. Factors likely to negatively impact on compliance included:

1. Regularly forgetting to take medications despite an intention to (14%).
2. Having trouble opening medication containers and/or swallowing tablets (15%).
3. Hoarding and using previously prescribed medication (35%).
4. Regularly altering dosages on the basis of symptomatic status (15%).
5. Reducing dosages to minimize costs (21%).

Conversely, identified factors likely to promote compliance included:

1. A belief that the medication regimen was either 'important or very important' for optimal management of the illness (85%).

2. A belief that the medication regimen was effective (64%).
3. Regularly attending the same medical clinic and pharmacy (94%).

Consequently, all HBI patients received a combination of remedial counselling, introduction of a compliance device/reminder routine and/or closer supervision by a caregiver (usually an immediate family member), and 37 patients (14%) were referred to their community pharmacist for more intensive follow-up thereafter. Most home visits lasted between 90 and 120 minutes.

Furthermore, all of the patients' primary care physicians were notified of this home assessment and any remedial action recommended: 40 patients (16%) were subject to immediate referral in order to address evidence of clinical deterioration and/or adverse effects of prescribed medication.

Primary end-point

The primary (composite) end-point occurred on 155 occasions in the HBI group and 217 occasions in the UC group ($p < 0.001$). This comprised 154 vs 197 unplanned readmissions ($p = 0.022$) and 1 vs 20 out-of-hospital deaths ($p < 0.001$, OR 0.04). The accumulated total of primary end-points during the six months of study follow-up are presented in Figure 5.2. It shows that the accumulation of primary end-points for the two groups was similar for the two groups in the initial 10 weeks of follow-up. Thereafter, the two groups continued to diverge in favour of the HBI group until the end of study follow-up at six months.

However, there was no significant difference in the number of patients in whom the primary end-point occurred (104 HBI vs 117 UC: $p = 0.299$), or in time

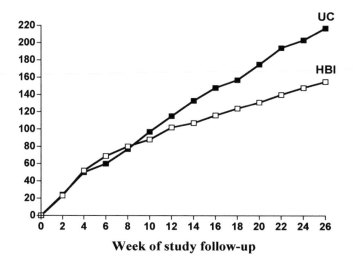

Figure 5.2: Accumulated total of unplanned readmissions plus out-of-hospital deaths during study follow-up according to study group.

to first readmission. Post hoc analysis of the frequency and characteristics of readmissions suggested that the major disparity occurred among patients who would normally experience multiple hospital admissions. Hence, the effect of the intervention was mediated through a difference in the frequency distribution of unplanned readmissions plus out-of-hospital deaths during study follow-up. Figure 5.3 represents the frequency of primary end-points during study follow-up according to study group. During study follow-up 12/103 HBI patients vs 24/105 UC patients (p = 0.035, OR 2.3) were readmitted on ≥ three occasions. In the UC group, patients with ≥ three readmissions were more likely to have a diagnosis of congestive heart failure (p < 0.001, OR 5.8) and/or chronic airways limitation (p = 0.005, OR 3.8), had experienced a previous unplanned admission within six months of the index admission (p = 0.005, OR 3.2) and were receiving a larger number of medications on discharge (mean 5.8 vs 4.6 medications per patient: p = 0.018).

Furthermore, blinded review of the medical records pertaining to all unplanned readmissions during study follow-up revealed that a greater proportion of UC admissions were associated with documented malcompliance and/or adverse effects of prescribed medication (35/197 vs 13/154: p = 0.012, OR 2.34).

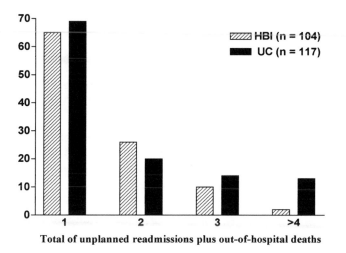

Figure 5.3: Frequency distribution of unplanned readmissions plus out-of-hospital deaths during study follow-up according to study group.

Secondary end-points

Total mortality was also significantly lower in the HBI group (12 vs 29: p = 0.006, OR 0.4). The Kaplan-Meier survival curves are presented in Figure 5.4. However, numbers of in-hospital deaths were similar for both groups (11 HBI vs 9 UC). Patient attendances at hospital emergency services were significantly lower in the

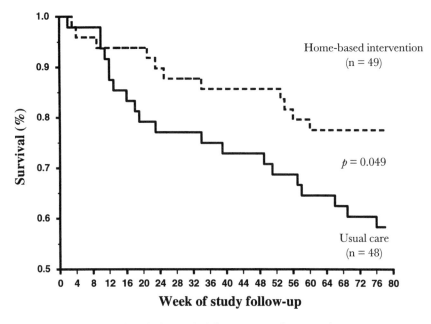

Figure 5.4: Cumulative survival during study follow-up according to study group.

HBI group (236 vs 314: $p < 0.001$), although the proportion of patients attending emergency services was similar (138 HBI vs 140 UC). Post-hoc analysis of the frequency of emergency service attendance suggested that patients in the UC group were more likely to attend emergency services ≥ three times during study follow-up (42/140 vs 18/138: $p < 0.001$, OR 2.9).

Total days of hospitalization resulting from *all* readmissions during study follow-up were significantly fewer in the HBI group (1452 vs 1766 days: $p < 0.001$). This comprised 1258 vs 1497 days associated with unplanned readmissions ($p < 0.001$) and 194 vs 269 days associated with elective admissions ($p < 0.001$).

Table 5.5 gives the results of univariate and subsequent multivariate analysis to determine significant correlates of unplanned readmission and out-of-hospital death. Adjusted odds ratios for relative probability of unplanned readmission in the entire study cohort were about 2.0 for patients with either prior dependence on home-based support or prior unplanned admission(s) and 2.2 for patients receiving ≥ five prescribed medications. Significant independent correlates for out-of-hospital death were non-English-speaking background and assignment to the UC group.

To determine whether there was significant interaction between treatment mode and correlates of unplanned readmission, multivariate analysis was also performed separately for each treatment group. In this respect there were no significant differences between treatments for identified correlates. The odds ratio for unplanned readmission during the study period was 3.2 (95% CI 1.4–7.6) for patients in the HBI group who were prospectively considered at high risk for readmission (n = 314) versus those considered at lower risk (n = 67). In the UC group, the corresponding odds ratio was 1.9 (95% CI 0.94–4.2).

Health-related quality of life

Quality-of-life scores indicated marked impairment of quality of life relative to age- and gender-matched norms for the local population for each of the eight health dimensions measured by the SF-36 as represented in Figure 5.5. However, there were no significant differences between the two groups, either at one or at three months after study entry (data not shown).

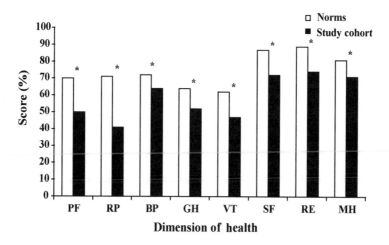

PF = physical functioning, RP = role functioning - physical, BP = bodily pain, GH = general health, V = vitality, SF = social functioning, RE = role functioning - emotional and MH = mental health*. All comparisons $p < 0.001$, Bonferroni test for multiple comparisons.

Figure 5.5: Comparison between SF-36 scores of study patients (n = 163) and age-matched and gender-matched SF-36 scores for the local population (n = 303).

Costs of health care

Costs of the two treatment regimens were compared for hospital-based health care in all patients, and community-based costs were estimated in a randomly chosen subset of 150 patients. Costs of hospital-based care tended to be lower among HBI patients with a mean of $2190 per patient versus $2680 per UC patient; this difference did not reach statistical significance ($p = 0.210$). On the other hand, the cost of implementing the study intervention among the 254 patients who received a home visit was $190 per patient (total $A48,460). Concerning community-based costs, no difference could be detected between groups as regards intensity of contact with primary care physicians (median of six consultations during study

Table 5.5: Results of univariate and subsequent multivariate analysis to determine significant correlates of unplanned readmission and out-of-hospital death.

Unplanned readmission	No (n = 554)	≥ 1 admission (n = 208)	*p* value Univariate analysis	Multivariate analysis	Adjusted odds ratio
Chronic illness at study entry	458 (83%)	186 (89%)	0.022	0.646	–
Age (mean ± SD)	65 ± 16	69 ± 15	0.003	0.143	–
Prior dependence on home support services	53 (9%)	44 (21%)	< 0.001	0.004	2.1 (1.2–3.1)
Number of prescribed discharge drugs (mean ± SD)	4.4 ± 2.5	5.6 ± 2.8	< 0.001	< 0.001	2.2* (1.6–3.1)
Emergency admission 6 months prior to study entry	394 (71%)	178 (86%)	< 0.001	< 0.001	2.1 (1.4–3.1)

Out-of-hospital death	No (741)	Yes (21)	*p* value Univariate analysis	Multivariate analysis	Adjusted odds ratio
Male	370 (50%)	14 (66%)	0.130	0.138	–
Emergency admission 6 months prior to study entry	156 (21%)	8 (38%)	0.100	0.929	–
Prescribed discharge medications (mean ± SD)	4.7 ± 2.6	5.5 ± 2.4	0.174	0.254	–
Initial medical admission	445 (60%)	17 (81%)	0.128	0.081	–
Primary language – non-English	84 (11%)	8 (38%)	0.002	< 0.001	4.7 (1.8–12)
Usual care post-hospitalization (UC group)	361 (49%)	20 (95%)	< 0.001	0.003	20.8 (2.7–156)

follow-up) or proportion of patients using home-based services (21% for both groups): mean cost of community-based care was \$610 per HBI patient versus \$630 per UC patient.

Effect of the study intervention among 'high-risk' patients with chronic heart failure

Rationale for a post-hoc subanalysis of outcomes associated with chronic heart failure

The largest clinical subgroup of patients involved in this study were patients with chronic heart failure. On the basis of the post-hoc analysis of the effects of HBI as regards a disproportionate reduction in recurrent readmissions to hospital and the evidence that patients with heart failure in particular are at risk of frequent hospital use and premature death, an intensive subset analysis was done on prospectively chosen high-risk patients with chronic congestive heart failure (n = 97). This subanalysis used the same end-points as for the overall cohort of patients in addition to a prospective analysis of the frequency distribution of all-cause unplanned admissions as well as those associated with acute heart failure. Furthermore, using additional clinical data specific to heart failure, multivariate analysis of clinical outcomes among this subset of patients was also performed.

Inclusion criteria for the subset analysis

Presence of chronic congestive heart failure was defined on the basis of formal demonstration (via echocardiography or radionuclide ventriculography) of impaired systolic function (left ventricular ejection fraction (LVEF) ≤ 55%) and persistent functional impairment indicative of New York Heart Association (NYHA) Class II, III or IV status. Acute heart failure was defined on the basis of pulmonary congestion/oedema evident on chest radiography[18], with a clinical syndrome of acute dyspnoea at rest. Chronicity of heart failure was diagnosed on the basis of exclusion of factors such as acute myocardial infarction or unstable angina pectoris that might have precipitated emergence of reduced systolic function at the time of index admission. However, patients admitted with acute ischaemia or infarction with previously documented heart failure were eligible for inclusion.

Randomization

Of the 107 eligible high-risk CHF patients initially identified, 97 (91%) agreed to participate in the study, with 48 patients assigned to UC and 49 patients assigned to HBI.

Results of subset analysis of patients with chronic heart failure

Clinical and demographic profile

Table 5.6 is a summary of the clinical and demographic profile of the study cohort. Consistent with the original cohort, most patients were older and of lower

Table 5.6: Baseline clinical and demographic data according to treatment group.

	HBI (n = 49)	UC (n = 48)
Demographic profile		
Male : Female	22 : 27	25 : 23
Age	76 ± 11 (40–93)	74 ± 10 (36–88)
Living alone	20	18
Non-English speaking background	10	10
Discharge medications		
Number of prescribed medications	6.9 ± 2.4 (2–15)	6.5 ± 2.5 (3–14)
Diuretic	49	47
ACE inhibitor	41	38
Digoxin	33	32
Nitrate	29	28
Warfarin	14	13
Hospitalization in the 6 months before the study		
Days of hospitalization prior to index admission	3.1 ± 5.8 (0–21)	3.2 ± 6.0 (0–24)
Duration of index admission (days)	7.9 ± 6.0 (2–27)	7.7 ± 6.2 (2–28)
CHF profile		
CHF documented prior to index admission	35	39
LVEF (%)	38 ± 11 (18–55)	39 ± 11 (17–55)
NYHA class II on discharge from hospital	24	24
NYHA class III	23	20
NYHA class IV	02	02
Comorbidity		
Ischaemic heart disease/myocardial infarction	35 : 20	30 : 21
Chronic airways limitation	21	14
Chronic hypertension	19	20
Atrial fibrillation	15	15
Non-insulin/insulin-dependent diabetes	7/2	10/2
Charlson Index of Co-morbidity	2.1 ± 0.7	2.2 ± 0.5
Admission profile		
Acute pulmonary oedema	30	27
Heart rate (beats/minute)	101 ± 24	94 ± 26
Systolic blood pressure (mm Hg)	138 ± 29	132 ± 27

Table 5.6: (contd).

	HBI (n = 49)	UC (n = 48)
Discharge profile		
Sodium mmol/L	138 ± 4.8	139 ± 3.4
Potassium mmol/L	4.0 ± 0.4	4.3 ± 0.5
Albumin g/L	39 ± 3.5	38 ± 4.3
Creatinine μmol/L	133 ± 43	150 ± 79
Heart rate (beats/minute)	79 ± 9	79 ± 13
Systolic blood pressure (mm Hg)	120 ± 21	120 ± 19
Sinus rhythm/Atrial fibrillation	31: 18	34 : 14

socio-economic status. Importantly, considering the potential for poorer health outcomes associated with suboptimal pharmacotherapy[19–23], all but one of the study cohort were prescribed a diuretic, 79 (81%) were given an angiotensin-converting enzyme inhibitor (ACE inhibitor) and 65 (67%) were given digoxin. However, probably because of the limited evidence at that time, few patients were prescribed a β-adrenoceptor blocker. Clinical data recorded at the time of index admission revealed that 57 (59%) patients were treated for acute pulmonary oedema and, of these, 16 (28%) had new onset of rapid uncontrolled (≥ 120 beats/minute) atrial fibrillation and 12 (21%) had an acute ischaemic syndrome: these data are consistent with those studies that show worsening cardiac function secondary to atrial fibrillation[24, 25] and/or acute myocardial ischaemia.[26] Also consistent with previous studies examining older cohorts of CHF patients, the extent and potential burden of comorbid illness(es) was great.[27]

Extent of study intervention

Consistent with the major cohort, seven HBI patients (14%) did not receive a home visit because of early readmission or withdrawal of consent. Among patients who were subject to a home visit, 22 (52%) were found to be malcompliant with their treatment regimen, and 38 (90%) had inadequate knowledge of their treatment regimen. On this basis, most patients needed remedial intervention during HBI, and nine patients were referred to a community pharmacist for more intensive follow-up. Furthermore, 14 (33%) patients showed early clinical deterioration and/or adverse effects from their medication regimen (most commonly postural hypotension in the presence of ACE inhibition) and needed immediate review by their primary care physician.

Primary end-point

During the study, the incidence of the primary composite end-point (unplanned readmission *plus* out-of-hospital death) was 0.76 vs 1.4 per HBI and UC patient respectively ($p = 0.03$). The accumulated totals of primary end-points are represented in Figure 5.6; as with the original study, the beneficial effects of HBI in this regard do not begin to become evident until the tenth week of follow-up. This comprised both fewer unplanned readmissions (36 vs 63; $p = 0.03$) and fewer out-of-hospital deaths (1 vs 5; $p = 0.11$) among HBI patients. There was no significant difference between groups with regard to time to first primary end-point, although HBI patients tended to be readmitted earlier.

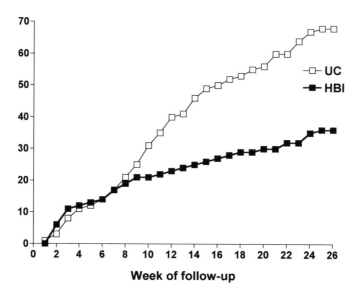

Figure 5.6: Accumulated total of unplanned readmissions plus out-of-hospital deaths during study follow-up.

Secondary end-points

Although fewer patients in the HBI group experienced an unplanned readmission (24/49 vs 31/38; $p = 0.12$) and/or died (6/49 vs 12/48; $p = 0.11$), neither difference reached statistical significance. Post-hoc analysis suggested that HBI was effective in preventing individual patients from requiring large numbers of readmissions with acute heart failure: no HBI patient had ≥ three such admissions, compared with five UC patients ($p = 0.02$). Patients assigned to HBI also recorded significantly fewer attendances at hospital emergency service (48 vs 87; $p = 0.05$) and fewer days of hospitalization (261 vs 452 days; $p = 0.05$).

Healthcare costs

The mean cost of hospital-based care tended to be lower for the HBI group ($3200) compared with the UC group ($5400); this difference did not reach statistical significance. On the other hand, the additional cost of implementing the study intervention was \$190 per patient. Costs associated with community-based health care for those patients subject to audit (n = 34) were similar for both groups: \$620 per HBI patient versus \$680 per UC patient.

Correlates of readmission and death

Correlates of readmission and death during the study are summarized in Table 5.7; both univariate and multivariate data are given. On multiple logistic regression, significant correlates of unplanned readmission were: 1) prolonged unplanned readmission prior to study entry, 2) living alone; and

Table 5.7: Correlates of unplanned readmission and mortality during study follow-up.

| Variable | Readmission | | p value | | |
	No (n = 42)	Yes (n = 55)	Univariate analysis	Multivariate analysis	Adjusted OR (95% CI)
Home-based intervention	31 (74%)	24 (44%)	0.12	0.06	0.4 (0.2–1.1)
Unplanned hospitalization ≤ 6 months before study (days)	8.1 ± 7.4	13.0 ± 8.9	0.005	0.002	5.2 (1.8–16.2)
Living alone	21 (50%)	37 (67%)	0.09	0.07	2.3* (0.9–5.7)
Prior admission for an acute ischaemic syndrome	25 (60%)	40 (73%)	0.2	0.02	3.3 (1.2–9.1)
Low albumin plasma concentration (g/L)	39 ± 3	37 ± 2	0.06	0.01	2.4* (1.2–6.0)

| Variable | Died | | p value | | |
	No (n = 79)	Yes (n = 18)	Univariate analysis	Multivariate analysis	Adjusted OR (95% CI)
Non-English-speaking background	11 (14%)	8 (44%)	< 0.001	< 0.001	5.0 (1.6–18)
Regular home support Services	23 (29%)	17 (94%)	< 0.001	0.03	15.7 (1.3–186)
Total readmissions during study follow-up	0.95 ± 1.4	1.9 ± 1.6	0.01	0.003	3.4* (1.3–11.2)

*Odds ratio shown for patients with ≥ 14 days of unplanned hospitalization, albumin plasma concentration of ≤ 38 g/L and ≥ two unplanned readmissions.

3) hypoalbuminaemia. Allocation to the UC regimen was a borderline correlate ($p = 0.06$). Significant correlates of mortality are: 1) non-English speaking, 2) regular home support; and 3) multiple readmissions during study follow-up.

An examination of the prolonged effects of the study intervention in the subset of patients with heart failure

Rationale

In the subset analysis of 'high-risk' patients with heart failure we showed that HBI was associated with reduced frequency of unplanned readmissions and fewer out-of-hospital deaths during 6 months follow-up. The apparent success of this strategy in reducing subsequent hospital use (42% in comparison with UC patients) was largely mediated through a reduction in recurrent admissions for acute heart failure. However, perhaps because of a combination of a small sample size, the skewed distribution of costs among UC patients and limited duration of follow-up, despite strong trends in favour of the study intervention we were unable to show definite cost savings or improved survival.

To examine the medium-term effects of the intervention on the original primary end-point and, more importantly, on frequency of recurrent hospital admissions, total hospital stay, cost of hospital-based care and total mortality, we extended follow-up of all surviving patients for a further 12 months (to a maximum of 18 months post index hospitalization for surviving patients).

Results of prolonged follow-up of patients with chronic heart failure

Primary end-point

During the 18 months following index hospitalization, 33/49 HBI patients (67%) versus 39/48 UC patients (81%) had experienced either an unplanned admission or an out-of-hospital death ($p = 0.12$). Although the two groups did not significantly differ with regard to the proportion of patients experiencing a primary end-point, patients in the HBI group accumulated significantly fewer unplanned readmissions (64 vs 125; $p = 0.02$) and suffered fewer out-of-hospital deaths (2 vs 9; $p = 0.02$; odds ratio 5.4). The combined total of primary end-points was therefore 66 vs 134 for the HBI and UC groups respectively (1.4 vs 2.7 events/patient: $p = 0.03$). Figure 5.7 shows that the two groups continued to diverge as regards accumulation of primary end-points (principally unplanned readmissions) during the additional 12 months of follow-up.

Secondary end-points

Overall, HBI patients required fewer days of hospitalization (both unplanned and elective) in comparison with UC patients (10.5 vs 21.1 days/patient;

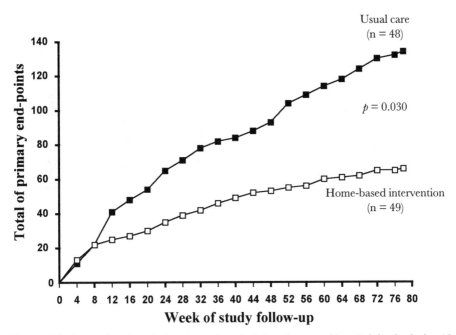

Figure 5.7: Accumulated total of unplanned readmission plus out-of-hospital deaths during 18 months follow-up.

$p = 0.02$) in addition to accumulating fewer attendances at the emergency department (2.5 vs 4.5 per patient; $p = 0.004$). On the basis of this reduction in hospital stay and comparable outpatient clinic costs, the calculated cost of hospital-based care per patient was significantly lower for the HBI group ($A5100 vs $A10,600; $p = 0.02$).

Analysis of the frequency distribution of unplanned readmissions showed that UC patients, once readmitted, were significantly more likely to experience $\geq$ four readmissions during study follow-up (12/38 vs 3/31; p = 0.03; odds ratio 4.2) whereas similar proportions of patients from the two groups were readmitted one, two and three times during study follow-up. Figure 5.8 shows the frequency distribution of unplanned readmissions for the two groups. Overall, 42% of all unplanned readmissions for the entire cohort were associated with a primary diagnosis of acute heart failure, the remainder being primarily associated with either an acute ischaemic syndrome or acute respiratory failure secondary to chronic airways limitation. Once readmitted, UC patients were significantly more likely to require $\geq$ three admissions for heart failure (8/21 vs 1/18; $p = 0.004$).

Patients assigned to HBI were also more likely to survive the 18-month period post index hospitalization: 11/49 HBI patients (20%) versus 20/48 UC patients (44%) died during follow-up ($p = 0.049$; odds ratio 0.41). Figure 5.9 represents the cumulative survival probability for the two study groups.

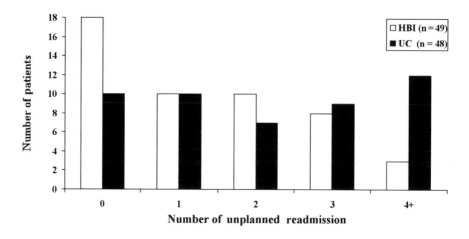

Figure 5.8: Frequency distribution of unplanned readmissions according to study group.

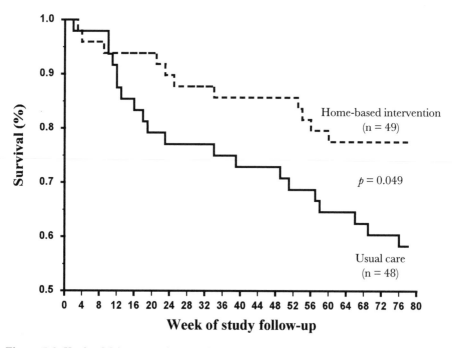

Figure 5.9: Kaplan-Meier curves for cumulative survival during 18-month follow-up (log-rank test for comparison of survival curves).

Correlates of unplanned readmission and mortality

On the basis of initial univariate analysis, the following variables were subjected to multiple logistic regression to determine potential correlates of unplanned readmission: previous admission(s) for acute heart failure, number of days of unplanned hospitalization in the six months *before* study follow-up, plasma albumin concentration on hospital discharge, NYHA class on hospital discharge and study group. Of these parameters, greater hospital use in the six months before study follow-up proved to be the only independent positive correlate of unplanned readmission in 18 months of index hospitalization. These data are summarized in Table 5.8.

Table 5.8: Correlates of unplanned readmission during 18-month follow-up.

| Variable | Unplanned readmission | | *p* value | | Adjusted OR (95% CI) |
	No (n = 28)	Yes (n = 69)	Univariate analysis	Multivariate analysis	
Unplanned days of hospitalization 6 months before study follow-up	6.8 ± 6.6	12.5 ± 8.8	0.002	0.006	5.4* (1.1–11.3)
Assignment to multidisciplinary, home-based intervention	18 (64%)	31 (45%)	0.08	0.09	0.5 (0.2–1.2)

*Adjusted odds ratio for ≥ 14 days unplanned hospitalization.

Similarly, the following variables were examined as potential correlates of mortality: duration of treatment for chronic heart failure, number of admissions for acute heart failure, number of days of unplanned hospitalization in the six months *before* study follow-up, LVEF, NYHA class on hospital discharge, English/non-English speaking background and study group. Of these parameters, greater hospital use in the six months before study follow-up, a non-English speaking background and lower LVEF were independent, positive correlates of 18-month mortality; conversely, assignment to HBI was a negative correlate. These data are summarized in Table 5.9.

Discussion

Overall beneficial effects of the study intervention

We initially examined the effect of a multidisciplinary, home-based intervention on the frequency of unplanned readmissions and out-of-hospital deaths among a heterogeneous cohort of largely frail and older patients requiring long-term medical care. In the six-month follow-up period, patients in the HBI group

Table 5.9: Correlates of unplanned readmission during 18-month follow-up.

| Variable | 18 month mortality | | *p* value | | Adjusted OR (95% CI) |
	No (n = 66)	Yes (n = 31)	Univariate analysis	Multivariate analysis	
Non-English speaking background	9 (14%)	12 (39%)	0.005	0.008	4.9 (1.5–15.4)
Days of unplanned hospitalization in the 6 months before follow-up	9.3 ± 7.4	14.4 ± 10.1	0.02	0.008	4.9* (1.6–15.2)
Assignment to multidisciplinary, home-based intervention	38 (59%)	11 (32%)	0.049	0.02	0.3 (0.1–0.82)
Left ventricular ejection fraction (%)	40.5 ± 10.7	34.9 ± 10.9	0.02	0.03	3.0** (1.1–8.6)

Adjusted odds ratio for * ≥ 14 days unplanned hospitalization and ** ≤ LVEF 40%.

showed a significant reduction in the primary end-point: a difference almost exclusively mediated by a reduction in multiple readmissions and out-of-hospital deaths. Although contact with primary care physicians and home-based services was similar for both groups, HBI patients had 18% fewer days of hospitalization. Examination of odds ratios for unplanned readmissions suggests that the 314 patients (82%) in the HBI group in whom the post-hospitalization intervention was performed constituted a well-delineated high-risk subset.

Potential mechanisms of beneficial effect

What are the potential explanations for these findings? As discussed in Chapter 4, studies have suggested that a significant proportion of unplanned hospital readmissions are preventable and that potentially avoidable causes of such readmissions include malcompliance with, and/or adverse effects of, prescribed medications, inadequate follow-up, suboptimal use of medical care and early clinical deterioration.[28] We postulated that the early HBI programme chosen might ameliorate all of the above factors, both directly and through increased vigilance of patients' physicians, community pharmacists and care-givers thereafter.

In this context, the study confirmed that one of the most important benefits of this type of HBI is the ability to obtain a more accurate picture of patients' management of their therapeutic regimen away from the artificial environment of the hospital. As such, the data obtained during the initial stage of the home visit provides clear evidence that the previously documented problems relating to suboptimal management of prescribed medications remain prevalent among those patients who can (theoretically) least afford to receive suboptimal treatment. Overall, the pattern of medication management was poor: many hitherto unknown and potentially serious problems were detected and this requires further comment.

Optimizing medication management[28]

Consistent with previous studies linking poorer compliance rates with chronic illness and/or greater number of prescribed medications[29-34], about half of the study cohort subjected to a 'reliable' pill count were found to be malcompliant, and those prescribed ≥ five medications had about a two-and-a-half-fold increased probability of significantly deviating from their planned treatment. Similarly, consistent with previous studies that have examined predominant areas of knowledge deficit in relation to prescribed medications[30, 35, 36], it was observed that although most patients (or relevant carers) were able to name the purpose, dosage and frequency of their prescribed medications, few were able to identify potential adverse effects and/or special instructions. On the basis of multivariate analysis, greater age, lower levels of formal education and presence of a chronic illness requiring treatment before the index admission were all independently associated with lower medication knowledge scores. While all of these parameters can probably be explained on the basis of a combination of reduced mental acuity and a lesser propensity to seek and absorb information, the absence of a relationship between medication compliance and knowledge (either on the basis of single knowledge items or the combined score) requires comment. Previous studies examining a potential relationship between the two have yielded conflicting results.[31, 35, 37, 38] There is, however, a compelling argument that greater knowledge does not necessarily lead to increased adherence to a regimen: it may in fact result in 'reasoned' non-compliance or there may simply be a deficit between behavioural intention and action, as was evident in a large number of the patients in the current study.[38, 39] In this context, the relative efficacy of strategies designed to directly improve compliance (for example, reminder cards and pre-packaging dosages) compared with those that aim to improve medication-related knowledge (for example, counselling) remains unknown. On a practical basis, it is probable that using a multifaceted approach (rather than a one-dimensional one) to address the 'multitude of sins' relating to the management of medications among the chronically ill is most likely to yield the best results.[40, 41] Unlike some previously reported studies[30, 42], and consistent with our previous observation that older patients with chronic illness have difficulty even remembering that they have received in-hospital counselling, [7] neither in-hospital self-medication nor incremental pre-discharge counselling (whether principally nurse-led or pharmacist-led) seemed to be associated with improved medication-related knowledge.

Similarly, on the basis of the 'reliable' pill counts we were unable to detect a modulating effect of these strategies on extent of compliance. However, consistent with other studies, potentially serious problems – including difficulty in opening medication containers[32, 43], hoarding of old medications, [31] and regularly altering dosages (often without informing the treating physician)[31, 37] – were detected during the home visit. As part of HBI all such problems were addressed through immediate intervention or incremental follow-up by the patient's GP or community pharmacist thereafter.

Because we chose to examine the effect of an intervention applied in the immediate post-discharge period, and any attempts to measure medication management in a similar fashion thereafter would have influenced the study outcome, we have no *direct* evidence of improved medication management following the HBI. However, the fact that this intervention was associated with reduced numbers of unplanned readmissions and improved survival suggests better use of prescribed medications was at least partially responsible for the improved health outcomes. Two components of post-hoc analysis of the original data in particular support this supposition. The first of these was blinded assessment of all unplanned readmissions during study follow-up. This revealed that a greater number of 'usual care' readmissions were related to documented malcompliance and/or adverse effects of prescribed medication. Of the 48 medication-related admissions identified, 34 (71%) were associated with adverse effects (ACE inhibitors being the most common precipitant in this regard) and 14 (29%) were associated with malcompliance. The other component of post-hoc analysis revealed that HBI was most effective in reducing recurrent unplanned readmissions among patients with chronic congestive heart failure.

Any interpretation of the medication-related data requires a caveat regarding the reliability and validity of the tools used to measure medication-related knowledge and compliance. Unfortunately, there is no 'gold-standard' measurement of medication compliance and all methods (including self-reporting, serial drug plasma concentration measurement and electronic container monitors) are fundamentally unreliable.[44, 45] However, it was anticipated that the pill counts used in the current study would be 'relatively' accurate on the following basis:

1. The number of pills dispensed at discharge was a known quantity.
2. There was a short period between dispensing of medications and the pill count.
3. Patients were unaware of the impending pill count.

Using a conservative approach, we accepted only those pill counts considered to be 'reliable' for any analysis of the data. This highlights the difficulties in accurately estimating compliance over even a short period of time, especially in the context of polypharmacy, and represents a caveat for the results of those studies measuring compliance in a similar context.

Similarly, the reliability, responsiveness and validity of the type of knowledge questionnaire used in this study (although widely used[30, 35]) must be questioned. In terms of 'reliability', we were able to eliminate the problem of inter-rater variation by employing one person (the study pharmacist) to assess patients using the same criterion for each medication. Furthermore, the composite knowledge scores for the entire cohort were near normally distributed. Although the questionnaire did not detect differences in knowledge components on the basis of in-hospital counselling and we did not measure changes over time, it did seem to be sensitive and therefore 'responsive' to the expected determinants of poorer knowledge. Furthermore, the components of medication-related knowledge tested are valid in that they are universally accepted as being essential to the optimal management of medications. However, does verbalization of information (for example, naming a potential adverse effect), representing a simple memory test, accurately reflect the depth of knowledge about a medication; especially if recall or recognition of an important piece of information about a medication is triggered only by an acute need (for example, actually experiencing an adverse effect)? It may have been possible to use more sophisticated tools to measure medication-related knowledge and behavioural intent, but in this largely frail and older cohort (including many from a non-English-speaking background) this would have been problematic.

Despite these potential limitations, the data relating to this cohort's management of their medication regimen highlight a number of important issues relevant to the apparent deficit between the 'potential' and 'actual' benefits of clinically 'proven' pharmacological agents. In this cohort of older, chronically ill patients, who would theoretically benefit most from appropriate and consistent treatment, medication management was often suboptimal. Hitherto unrecognized problems were many and varied among the study cohort, with malcompliance probably representing the most significant of these (especially in the presence of minimal medication-related knowledge and multiple disease states) and the problem most likely to result in poorer health outcomes. Importantly, for this cohort at least, in-hospital counselling was not associated with either improved compliance or medication knowledge. However, consistent with previous reports of this type of intervention[46], HBI was responsible for the detection of many hitherto unknown problems and was associated with an overall reduction in readmissions; in particular those associated with either known malcompliance and/or adverse effects of the prescribed regimen.

Recurrent unplanned readmissions

Despite the reduction in total unplanned readmissions in the HBI group, the proportion of patients readmitted at six months was similar in both groups. The beneficial effect of the study intervention seemed to be confined largely to the subgroup of patients who would usually be at risk of multiple unplanned readmissions and out-of-hospital death. It was noted as a component of post-hoc analysis that the frequency of distribution of numbers of readmissions differed significantly between UC and HBI groups, with a disproportionately low number of multiple readmissions in the HBI group. Coupled with the analysis of predictors of three or more readmissions among UC patients, these data suggest that the predominant benefit of HBI may lie in patients at particular risk of multiple readmissions. This is not unprecedented for this type of HBI as both Townsend et al. (1988)[47] and Rich et al. (1995)[13] have shown that interventions involving a component of home visits reduce the frequency of multiple readmissions to hospital.

Comparison with other studies

Although a number of previous investigations have sought to reduce frequency of readmissions to hospital, through both community and hospital-based strategies [11, 13, 48–60], the current methodology differs from such studies with its use of an HBI to both identify and correct medication-related problems and increase caregiver vigilance thereafter. As discussed earlier, two previously reported studies of HBI involving non-medical personnel have had some success in reducing rates of readmissions, respectively after 18 months in a study of patients with a wide range of chronic illnesses[47], and (most notably) after three months in patients with chronic congestive heart failure.[13] The results of the current study and the two previous studies are to some extent consistent with the findings of a meta-analysis of randomized controlled studies examining the value of geriatric assessment programmes. On the basis of this analysis, Stuck and colleagues (1993) concluded that such programmes are associated with a 12% risk reduction in readmission during study follow-up.[61] However, the current study differs from those used in the meta-analysis in that it involves a more transient and potentially more cost-effective intervention, and reports a significant reduction in mortality associated with a post-discharge intervention; previously reported reductions in mortality have been primarily associated with hospital-based interventions and patient cohorts discharged to home or long-term institutional care.[61–63]

Selection of 'high risk' patients with chronic heart failure for subset analysis

On the basis of the original analysis of the major cohort, comprising both cardiac and non-cardiac patients, and the positive results reported by Rich et al.[13] relating to a similar intervention specifically targeting 'high-risk' patients with chronic congestive heart failure, we postulated that this intervention would be particularly effective in reducing recurrent readmissions of such patients. In selecting relatively higher risk patients with heart failure (patients had already been selected on the basis of greater risk because of the presence of a chronic illness) we prospectively identified two important determinants for increased risk for hospital readmission and premature death – prior hospitalization for acute heart failure and functional impairment refractory to pharmacotherapy.[64, 65] Furthermore, although the extent of left ventricular systolic dysfunction, as determined by measurement of the left ventricular ejection fraction, has not been shown to be consistently predictive or associated with increased hospital use or premature death[66], we chose to include only those patients with at least some left ventricular systolic dysfunction. At the very least, this ensured that the patient cohort was homogeneous as regards baseline, demographic and clinical characteristics and prescribed pharmacotherapy, and the rate of subsequent morbidity and mortality was certainly high during study follow-up.

Beneficial effects of the intervention among patients with chronic heart failure

The subanalysis showed that during study follow-up, patients with chronic heart failure randomized to HBI had significantly fewer unplanned readmissions and out-of-hospital deaths. Despite the greater number of deaths in the UC group (and hence no further potential for admission), there was still a 42% difference in overall duration of hospital stay. The overall improvement in health outcomes among HBI patients is consistent with the degree of intervention during, and subsequent to, the home visit. Many of the problems uncovered during this visit would have hitherto remained undetected. Analysis of the pattern and potential predictors of an unplanned readmission suggests that this type of HBI is most effective among patients with problems that contribute to poor control of their heart failure, resulting in multiple readmissions – especially if they have more severe systolic dysfunction and/or less social support. There was also a trend towards fewer out-of-hospital deaths among HBI patients.

Specific comparison with other studies of patients with chronic heart failure

At the time these studies were completed (1999) there were four other randomized controlled investigations that had also included high proportions of patients with heart failure. Two of these studies involved 'broad' interventions (comprehensive discharge planning[55] and increased access to outpatient primary care[59]) and yielded inconclusive and unfavourable results respectively, in relation to extent and duration of rehospitalization. In two other studies, however, use of similar but more intensive interventions specific to management of chronic heart failure were associated with a significant increase in the time to first readmission or out-of-hospital death at three months post-discharge among 'high-risk' patients with heart failure from a hospital in the US[13], and delayed readmission and trends towards reduced hospitalization and costs at one year among a relatively non-selected cohort of patients with heart failure from a hospital in Malmö, Sweden.[58]

As with the study we had undertaken, the difference between groups as regards frequency of readmissions in the study reported by Rich and colleagues (1995) was largely mediated through fewer multiple readmissions in patients exposed to the nurse-directed, multidisciplinary intervention incorporating home visits.[13] It is possible that the success of the regimen examined in this study may have resulted from a combination of a home visit (a central component of the approach used by Rich et al.) and a broad-based examination of chronic morbidity. As expected[64, 65], just under half of all readmissions were primarily associated with a co-morbid condition. This is not surprising considering the significant co-morbidity present in this cohort. In a similar cohort of patients with heart failure, Blyth and colleagues (1997) noted a seasonal pattern of increased admissions owing to respiratory failure[67], an observation confirmed by French national data.[68]

One explanation for the results of this study might be that UC patients received inadequate care relative to currently established norms for the management of chronic heart failure, resulting in a higher incidence of readmission and mortality. However, clinical data, pharmacotherapy and morbidity were all similar to data for analogous groups in contemporary publications[64, 65, 67] and guidelines for the management of heart failure.[69] In a multicentre study of hospital readmissions and mortality among a broad population of patients with chronic heart failure in the US, the six-monthly rates of readmission and mortality were reported to be 44% and 24% respectively.[64] In this study, the proportion of UC patients readmitted at six months was not unexpectedly higher (65%), and mortality was similar (25%).

Correlates of unplanned readmission

A number of the correlates of unplanned readmission among this subset of patients are consistent with those in previous studies. As expected, greater hospital use prior to study follow-up, even when potentially confounded by more parameters specific to heart failure, was a powerful predictor for subsequent hospitalization.[70-72] Similarly, the other correlates of readmission have been previously correlated with poorer health outcomes. These included a prior hospitalization associated with an acute ischaemic syndrome[72, 73], hypoalbuminaemia[74], and living alone.[7, 75]

Prolonged beneficial effects of multidisciplinary, home-based intervention among patients with chronic heart failure

Although the subset analysis of patients with chronic heart failure revealed particular benefits in respect of extent and duration of readmission, perhaps because of a combination of a small sample size, the skewed distribution of costs among UC patients and limited duration of follow-up, analysis of six-month data showed neither definite cost savings nor improved survival. The prolonged follow-up of this cohort of patients was therefore undertaken to determine whether there was any marked accentuation or attenuation of beneficial effects of HBI in the medium term. In this respect, the results of the extended follow-up showed continued benefit with regard to the primary end-point of frequency of unplanned readmissions plus out-of-hospital death; HBI patients accumulated about 50% fewer end-points. The data also suggested that the two groups continued to diverge for accumulation of these end-points in the 12–18 months following the single home visit (see Figure 4.7). While there was a trend towards fewer HBI patients requiring an unplanned readmission during study follow-up (31/49 vs 38/48; $p = 0.08$), the continued differential between groups for accumulating unplanned readmissions potentially reflects the selective effect of HBI on patients otherwise likely to have frequent, recurrent unplanned readmissions. Rich et al. also reported that post-hoc analysis of the effects of a similar, but more intensive, intervention that was implemented for three months after discharge suggested that the beneficial effects of the intervention lasted up to a year, although it is not clear whether this was mediated through a sustained reduction in multiple readmissions among intervention patients.[13]

With larger numbers of patients needing hospitalization during the extended follow-up, the skewness and variability of accumulated costs were less accentuated and we were able to show that the approximate 50% reduction in hospital stay among HBI patients translated to a significant reduction in hospital-based costs of a similar magnitude. Once again, however, the subset of patients needing repeated readmissions contributed disproportionately to the overall costs for their respective groups. This is consistent with the existence of so-called 'high-cost' users whose repeated admissions for acute exacerbations of a chronic illness cost far more than single, high-cost admissions.[76, 77]

Although the difference in group mortality rates just reached statistical significance, the magnitude of the apparent reduction in mortality among HBI patients was large (about 50%) and multivariate analysis showed a stronger relationship between assignment to HBI and survival. In our original analysis, out-of-hospital death was included in the primary end-point to partially adjust for the fact that patients would no longer need hospital admission. However, the frequency of out-of-hospital death alone has proved to be far greater than expected, with significantly more of these events occurring among UC patients, both at six months in the original heterogeneous cohort of hospitalized patients, and at 18 months among this subset of patients; proving to be the primary difference in both cases for the reduced overall mortality among HBI patients.

Specific comparison with other studies of patients with chronic congestive heart failure

Such a proportional improvement in survival rates (if verified) in larger studies would be more than comparable with those reported in the original (and larger) ACE inhibitor trials.[78] The 18-month mortality rate among the UC group in this study was somewhat greater than that reported in more recent clinical trials that have included carefully selected patients with heart failure receiving ACE inhibitors as standard therapy and generally lower LVEFs.[79] However, the survival profile of UC patients in the current study, at both 6 and 18 months, is comparable to that reported at 6 and 12 months among similar cohorts of hospitalized patients with heart failure.[64, 65, 67]

Changing determinants of outcome during prolonged follow-up

After 18 months of more extended follow-up the only consistent independent determinant of unplanned readmission was greater hospital use before study follow-up. Therefore the other correlates of six-month unplanned readmission, living alone, prior admission for an acute ischaemic syndrome and hypoalbuminaemia, were no longer predictive of such outcomes. Although it is inherently difficult in these circumstances (that is, in a relatively small cohort of patients) to reliably identify determinants of outcome, the emergence of prior hospitalization as a consistent and robust predictor of subsequent hospitalization, as has been discussed previously, was not unexpected, especially considering the relative contribution (potentially 60% or more) of other chronic disease states. However, consistent with previous studies, greater functional impairment as determined by NYHA class on discharge from index hospitalization was, on univariate analysis, significantly associated with subsequent readmission and was the last parameter to be step-wise rejected in the multiple logistic regression model.[64–67, 72] Although this is not surprising, considering the fluctuations in clinical response to therapeutics among patients with heart failure and the subjective nature of assessing patients in this manner, the fact that functional impairment seemed to be more predictive of readmission than the patient's documented LVEF is consistent with results of previously reported studies.[64–67, 72] This probably reflects the fact that these two parameters have been rarely shown to be correlated[66] and that the extent of functional impairment is more likely to be sensitive to both left ventricular systolic and diastolic dysfunction and the influence of suboptimal treatment with regard to hospital admissions.

Patients with greater hospital use in the six months before study follow-up also had poorer survival rates. The fact that the improved survival associated with HBI was independent of the most proven and reliable predictor of poorer health outcomes among the chronically ill is reassuring. The only independent correlate of mortality specific to chronic heart failure was a relatively lower LVEF; patients with a LVEF ≤ 40% had an approximate three-fold increased probability of dying during 18-month follow-up. Although left ventricular ejection fraction has not been proved to be a reliable predictor of mortality in some studies (possibly because of measurement variability[66] and the influence of ventricular interaction during diastole[80–82]), these data are consistent with a recently reported large study of a similar cohort of patients with chronic heart failure in the US, which also showed that more severe systolic dysfunction is associated with poorer survival.[65]

Potential reasons for prolonged beneficial effects

Many forms of therapeutic intervention (including non-pharmacological interven-tion) have been shown to be highly effective for a short period of time but to have no significant beneficial impact beyond the first few days or weeks after withdrawal of the therapeutic agent.[82] How and why is it possible for a single post-hospitalization intervention to continue to exert a beneficial effect on readmissions and mortality for at least 18 months after implementation? As discussed earlier, we anticipated that an early post-hospitalization HBI would not only be beneficial in detecting clinical deterioration likely to lead to short-term hospital readmission(s), but would detect hitherto unrecognized problems likely to contribute to poorer longer-term outcomes. Although we have no direct evidence of mechanisms of beneficial effect of the current HBI, the magnitude of problems detected during the home visit that required remedial action (many of which have been identified previously as contributing to unplanned hospitalization – for example, malcompliance with and/or adverse effects of treatment regimen, early clinical deterioration and subop-timal use of medical care especially among non-English-speaking patients) is consis-tent with two previous reports on the mechanisms of the beneficial effect of interventions that involve a home visit.[13, 46] In respect to improved survival, it is possible that a combination of increased vigilance of carers, improved compliance and increased awareness of the therapeutic goals of treatment and better use of available medical care among HBI patients led to a reduced incidence of acute deterioration and death before hospital care could be accessed. It is important to note that although the study intervention seems to be limited (that is, confined to the period immediately after discharge), the potential for changes in the long-term structure of health care – through the patient's pharmacist, general practitioner, community nurse and/or cardiologist hospital, and stimulated by the initial detec-tion and reporting of previously undetected problems – quite probably contributed to the prolonged beneficial effects of the intervention. However, the precise mechan-ism(s) of the beneficial effect of the HBI in this regard is unlikely to be elucidated.

Study limitations

This study had several limitations, including (as discussed above) lack of clear identification of mechanism(s) of beneficial effect and limited duration of follow-up. In the study 82% of patients randomized to HBI were categorized as high-risk and therefore received in-hospital and home-based components of intervention. It therefore remained uncertain whether the in-hospital component of intervention (counselling by a pharmacist and/or study nurse) contributed to the overall benefi-cial effect of HBI, despite the data that suggested that this component was not associated with a noticeable improvement in medication management. Furthermore, the results of the study may be applicable only to patients of similar socio-economic status to those investigated.

Such limitations also apply to the additional analysis of the 'high-risk' patients with heart failure, who represented a subset of the total trial population. The fact that we were unable to propose the exact mechanism(s) of beneficial effect of HBI even among the more comprehensively characterized cohort of patients with heart failure reflects the minimalistic nature of the study. This problem is, however, common to other interventions incorporating a multifaceted approach. The subanalysis of the outcomes of patients with chronic heart failure was also limited by the size of this cohort of patients in the study; hence the need to extend study follow-up to examine less frequently occurring end-points (for example, mortality). Furthermore, we had no data on functional status and quality of life among surviving patients.

Summary

In our initial study *we** showed that an inexpensive and essentially transient HBI reduces unplanned readmissions and mortality among a large, heterogeneous cohort of predominantly older cardiac and non-cardiac patients discharged home after acute hospitalization. The subsequent analysis of the effects of the intervention among the limited number of 'high-risk' patients with chronic congestive heart failure participating in the study (representing a group of patients most vulnerable to often preventable factors leading to increased frequency of hospitalization) suggested that this type of intervention would be particularly cost-effective if applied selectively to similar patients in the future. This was further supported by data from the extended follow-up of such patients, which showed prolonged benefits in subsequent hospitalization and mortality: to our knowledge this represents the first report of a non-pharmacological intervention of this type improving survival among hospitalized patients with heart failure while significantly reducing hospital readmissions.

At this stage of our investigations it was appropriate, however, to perform a sufficiently powered randomized controlled study of this type of intervention targeting a similar cohort of 'high-risk' patients with heart failure that looked at a number of residual issues not adequately addressed by the current study. These included the following key issues:

Which component of the intervention used in the current study (in-hospital counselling or home visits and subsequent arrangement of more intensive follow-up thereafter) was most effective in reducing subsequent unplanned readmissions and out-of-hospital deaths, or does this intervention rely on a synergy between the two components of intervention?

---

*The *we* in relation to this research programme refers, to a large extent, to Sue Pearson, who made a significant contribution to the original design of the study and undertook many of the home visits as part of the study intervention. It also refers to Professor John Horowitz, who provided a healthy dose of critical thought and analysis after the initial study had been performed.

Similarly, is it necessary (particularly in the context of minimizing the cost of an intervention) to use both a pharmacist and a nurse to visit chronic heart failure patients, if an appropriately qualified cardiac nurse is able to deal with medication-related issues?

In this respect, would a more heart failure-specific intervention be more effective than the broad intervention used in the current study? For example, it seemed logical to include more specific components of education with regard to optimal diet, fluid management and exercise for patients with heart failure. Strict exercise regimens in particular have been shown to have beneficial effects in younger patients with heart failure[83, 84], and although the type of cohort included in this study would be unlikely to tolerate such programmes, those programmes that have specifically targeted older patients have also shown some benefits.[85]

Would the intervention be more effective if home visits were selectively repeated among patients who show recurrent readmissions despite initial intervention?

What are some of the measurable mechanisms of beneficial effect of this type of intervention?

Assuming the intervention is associated with prolonged survival (at least in the short term to medium term) what are its effects on subsequent functional status and health-related quality of life among surviving patients?

If the efficacy of this relatively novel approach to managing high-risk patients with heart failure was confirmed in a prospective randomized controlled trial, it would represent an attractive and relatively cheap means to both improve health outcomes among such patients and deliver significant cost savings.

References

1. Stewart S, Pearson S, Luke CG, et al. Effects of a home-based intervention on unplanned readmissions and out-of-hospital deaths. *J Am Geriatr Soc* 1998; 46: 174–80.
2. Stewart S, Pearson S, Horowitz JD. Effects of a home-based intervention among congestive heart failure patients discharged from acute hospital care. *Arch Intern Med* 1998; 158: 1067–72.
3. Stewart S, Vandenbroek AJ, Pearson S, et al. Prolonged beneficial effects of a home-based intervention on unplanned readmissions and mortality among congestive heart failure patients. *Arch Intern Med* 1999; 159: 257–61.
4. Mathers C. *Health Differentials Among Adult Australians Aged 25–64 Years.* Canberra: Australian Institute of Health and Welfare: Health Monitoring Series No.1. Australian Government Publishing Service, 1994.
5. Glover J, Sharnd M, Foster C, et al. *A Social Health Atlas of South Australia* (2nd edition). Adelaide: Policy and Budget Division, South Australian Health Commission, 1996.
6. Charlson ME, Pompei P, Ales KL, et al. A new method of classifying prognostic comorbidity in longitudinal studies: Development and validation. *J Chron Dis* 1987; 40: 373–83.
7. Stewart S, Davey M, De-Sanctis M, et al. Home medication management: A study of patients post-hospitalisation. *Australian Pharmacist* 1995; 4: 472–6.
8. Anderson GF, Steinberg EP. Hospital readmissions in the Medicare population. *N Engl J Med* 1984; 311: 1349–53.

9.   Victor CR, Vetter NJ. The early readmission of the elderly to hospital. *Age and Ageing* 1985; 14: 37–42.

10.   Fethke CC, Smith IM, Johnson N. Risk factors affecting readmission of the elderly into the health care system. *Med Care* 1986; 24: 427–37.

11.   Evans RL, Hendricks RD, Lawrence KV, et al. Identifying factors associated with health care use: A hospital-based screening index. *Soc Scient Med* 1988; 27: 947–54.

12.   Williams IE, Fitton F. Factors affecting early unplanned readmission of elderly patients to hospital. *BMJ* 1988; 297: 784–7.

13.   Rich MW, Beckham V, Wittenberg C, et al. A multidisciplinary intervention to prevent the readmission of elderly patients with congestive heart failure. *New Engl J Med* 1995; 333: 1190–5.

14.   McCallum J. The SF-36 in an Australian sample: Validation. *Aust J Public Health* 1995; 19: 160–6.

15.   McHorney C, Ware J, Raczek A. The MOS 36-item short form health survey (SF-36): Psychometric and clinical tests of validity in measuring physical and mental health constructs. *Med Care* 1994; 32: 551–67.

16.   Ware J, Sherbourne C. The MOS 36-item short-form health survey (SF-36): Conceptual framework and item selection. *Med Care* 1992; 30: 473–83.

17.   Watson E, Firman D, Baade P, et al. Telephone administration of the SF-36 health survey: Validation studies and population norms for adults in Queensland. *Aust NZ J Public Health* 1996; 20: 359–63.

18.   Mahydoon R, Klein RK, Jeffrey WE, et al. Radiographic pulmonary congestion in end-stage congestive heart failure. *Am J Cardiol* 1989; 63: 625–7.

19.   Reis SE, Holubkov R, Edmundowicz D, et al. Treatment of patients admitted to hospital with congestive heart failure: Specialty-related disparities in practice patterns and outcomes. *J Am Coll Cardiol* 1997; 30: 733–8.

20.   Pearson TA, Peters TD. The treatment gap in coronary artery disease and heart failure: Community standards and the post-discharge patient. *Am J Cardiol* 1997; 80(suppl): 45H–52H.

21.   Smith N, Psaty B, Pitt B, et al. Temporal patterns in the medical treatment of congestive heart failure with angiotensin-converting enzyme inhibitors in older adults, 1989 through 1995. *Arch Intern Med* 1998; 158: 1081–98.

22.   Edep ME, Shah NB, Tateo IM, et al. Difference between primary care physicians and cardiologists in management of congestive heart failure: Relation to practice guidelines. *J Am Coll Cardiol* 1997; 30: 518–26.

23.   Stafford RS, Saglam D, Blumenthal D. National patterns of angiotensin-converting enzyme inhibitor use in congestive heart failure. *Arch Intern Med* 1997; 157: 2460–4.

24.   Crijns HJ, Van den Berg MP, Van Gelder IC, et al. Management of atrial fibrillation in the setting of heart failure. *Eur Heart J* 1997; 18: C45–9.

25.   Van den Berg MP, Tuinenburg AE, Crijns HJ, et al. Heart failure and atrial fibrillation: Current concepts and controversies. *Heart* 1997; 77: 309–13.

26.   Goldberger MJ, Peled HB, Stroh JA, et al. Prognostic factors in acute pulmonary edema. *Arch Intern Med* 1986; 146: 489–93.

27.   Brown A, Cleland J. Influence of concomitant disease on patterns of hospitalization in patients with heart failure discharged from Scottish hospitals in 1995. *Eur Heart J* 1998; 19: 1063–9.

28.   Stewart S, Davey M, Desanctis M, et al. Home medication management: A study of patient post-hospitalisation. *Australian Pharmacist* 1995; 14: 472–6.

29. Wright E. Non-compliance – or how many aunts has Matilda? *Lancet* 1993; 342: 909–13.
30. Lowe CJ, Raynor DK, Courtney EA, et al. Effects of self medication programme on knowledge of drugs and compliance with treatment in elderly patients. *BMJ* 1995; 310: 1229–31.
31. Parkin D, Henney C, Quirk J, et al. Deviation from prescribed drug treatment after discharge from hospital. *BMJ* 1976; 2: 686–8.
32. Nikolaus T, Kruse W, Bach M, et al. Elderly patients' problems with medication. An in-hospital and follow-up study. *Euro J Clin Pharmacol* 1996; 49: 255–9.
33. Graveley EA, Oseasohn CS. Multiple drug regimens: Medication compliance among veterans 65 years and older. *Research in Nursing and Health* 1991; 14: 51–8.
34. Coons SJ, Sheahan SL, Martin SS, et al. Predictors of medication noncompliance in a sample of older adults. *Clin Ther* 1994; 16: 110–17.
35. Furlong S. Do programmes of medicine self-administration enhance patient knowledge, compliance and satisfaction? *J Adv Nurs* 1996; 23: 1254–62.
36. Veggeland T, Fagerheim KU, Ritland T, et al. Do patients know enough about their medication? A questionnaire among cardiac patients discharged from 5 Norwegian hospitals. *Tidsskrift for Den Norske Laegeforening* 1993; 113: 3013–16.
37. Donovan J, Blake D. Patient non-compliance: Deviance or reasoned decision-making? *Soc Sci Med* 1992; 34: 507–13.
38. McMahon T, Clark C, Bailie G. Who provides patients with drug information? *BMJ* 1987; 294: 355–6.
39. Conrad P. The meaning of medications: Another look at compliance. *Soc Sci Med* 1985; 20: 29–37.
40. Miller N, Hill M, Kottke T, et al. The multilevel compliance challenge: Recommendations for a call to action. *Circulation* 1997; 95: 1085–90.
41. Haynes BR, Taylor WD, Sackett DL. *Compliance in Health Care.* Baltimore, MD: Johns Hopkins University Press, 1979.
42. Pereles L, Romonko L, Murzyn T, et al. Evaluation of a self-medication program. *J Am Geriatr Soc* 1996; 44: 161–5.
43. Blenkiron P. The elderly and their medication: Understanding and compliance in a family practice. *Postgrad Med J* 1996; 72: 671–6.
44. Cargill JM. Medication compliance in elderly people: Influencing variables and intervention. *J Adv Nursing* 1992; 17: 422–6.
45. Cramer JA. Microelectronic systems for monitoring and enhancing patient compliance with medication regimens. *Drugs* 1995; 3: 321–7.
46. Alessi CA, Stuck AE, Aronow HU, et al. The process of care in preventive in-home comprehensive geriatric assessment. *J Am Geriatr Soc* 1997; 45: 1044–50.
47. Townsend J, Piper M, Frank AO, et al. Reduction in hospital readmission stay of elderly patients by a community based hospital discharge scheme: A randomised controlled trial. *BMJ* 1988; 297: 544–7.
48. Winograd CH, Gerety MB, Lai NA. A negative trial of inpatient geriatric consultation. *Arch Intern Med* 1993; 153: 2017–23.
49. Melin A, Bergin L. Efficacy of the rehabilitation of elderly primary care patients after short-stay hospital treatment. *Med Care* 1995; 30: 1004–15.
50. Thomas DR, Brahan R, Haywood BP. Inpatient community-based geriatric assessment reduces subsequent mortality. *J of Am Geriatr Soc* 1993; 41: 101–4.
51. Hansen FR, Spedtsberg K, Schroll M. Geriatric follow-up by home visits after discharge from hospital: A randomized controlled trial. *Age and Ageing* 1992; 21: 445–50.

52. Rubin CD, Sizemore MT, Loftis PA, et al. The effect of geriatric evaluation and management on Medicare reimbursement in a large public hospital: A randomized clinical trial. *J Am Geriatr Soc* 1992; 40: 989–95.

53. Siu AL, Kravitz RL, Keeler E, et al. Postdischarge geriatric assessment of hospitalized frail elderly patients. *Arch Intern Med* 1996; 156: 76–81.

54. Fitzgerald JF, Smith DM, Martin DK, et al. A case manager intervention to reduce readmissions. *Arch Intern Med* 1994; 154: 1721–9.

55. Naylor M, Brooten D, Jones R, et al. Comprehensive discharge planning for the hospitalized elderly. *Ann Intern Med* 1994; 120: 999–1006.

56. Naylor MD, Brooten D, Cambell R, et al. Comprehensive discharge planning and home follow-up of hospitalized elders: A randomized clinical trial. *JAMA* 1999; 281: 613–20.

57. Smith DM, Weinberger M, Katz BP, et al. Post discharge care and readmissions. *Med Care* 1988; 26: 699–708.

58. Cline C, Israelsson B, Willenheimer R, et al. A cost effective management programme for heart failure reduces hospitalisation. *Heart* 1998; 80: 442–6.

59. Weinberger M, Oddone EZ, Henderson WG. Does increased access to primary care reduce hospital readmissions? *New Engl J Med* 1996; 334: 1441–7.

60. Jaarsma T, Halfens R, Huijer Abu-Saad H, et al. Effects of education and support on self-care and resource utilization in patients with heart failure. *Eur Heart J* 1999; 20: 673–82.

61. Stuck AE, Siu AL, Wieland DG, et al. Comprehensive geriatric assessment: A meta-analysis of controlled trials. *Lancet* 1993; 342: 1032–6.

62. Rubenstein LZ, Josephson KR, Wieland DG, et al. Effectiveness of a geriatric evaluation unit: A randomized clinical trial. *New Engl J Med* 1984; 311: 1664–70.

63. Thomas DR, Brahan R, Haywood BP. Inpatient community-based geriatric assessment reduces subsequent mortality. *J Am Geriatr Soc* 1993; 41: 101–4.

64. Krumholz HM, Parent EM, Tu N, et al. Readmission after hospitalisation for congestive heart failure among Medicare beneficiaries. *Arch Intern Med* 1997; 157: 99–104.

65. Jaagosild P, Dawson N, Thomas C, et al. Outcomes of acute exacerbation of severe congestive heart failure. *Arch Intern Med* 1998; 158: 1081–9.

66. Cowburn P, Cleland J, Coats A, et al. Risk stratification in chronic heart failure. *Eur Heart J* 1998; 19: 696–710.

67. Blyth F, Lazarus R, Ross D, et al. Burden and outcomes of hospitalization for congestive heart failure. *MJA* 1997; 167: 67–70.

68. Boulay F, Berthier F, Sisteron O, et al. Seasonal variation in chronic heart failure hospitalizations and mortality in France. *Circulation* 1999; 3: 280–6.

69. The ACC/AHA Task Force on Practice Guidelines (Committee on Evaluation and Management of Heart Failure). Guidelines for the evaluation and management of heart failure. *J Am Coll Card* 1995; 26: 1376–98.

70. Graham H, Livesley B. Can readmissions to a geriatric medical unit be prevented. *Lancet* 1983; i: 404–6.

71. Ashton CM, Kuykendall DH, Johnson ML, et al. The association between quality of inpatient care and early readmission. *Ann Intern Med* 1995; 122: 415–21.

72. Vinson JM, Rich MW, Sperry JC, et al. Early readmission of elderly patients with congestive heart failure. *J Am Geriatr Soc* 1990; 38: 1290–5.

73. Chin MH, Goldman L. Correlates of major complications or death in patients with patients admitted to the hospital with congestive heart failure. *Arch Intern Med* 1996; 156: 1814–20.

74. Hermann FR, Safran C, Levkoff SE, et al. Serum albumin level on admission as a predictor of death, length of stay and readmission. *Arch Intern Med* 1992; 152: 125–30.

75. Bigby JA, Dunn J, Goldman L, et al. Assessing the preventability of emergency hospital admissions. *Am J Med* 1987; 83: 1031–6.

76. Anderson GF, Steinberg EP. Hospital readmissions in the Medicare population. *N Engl J Med* 1984; 311: 1349–53.

77. Zook CJ, Moore FD. High-cost users of medical care. *N Engl J Med* 1980; 302: 996–1002.

78. The CONSENSUS Trial Study Group. Effects of enalapril on mortality in severe congestive heart failure: Results of the Cooperative North Scandinavian Enalapril Survival Study (CONSENSUS). *N Engl J Med* 1987; 316: 1429–35.

79. Petrie M, Berry C, Stewart S, et al. Failing ageing hearts. *Eur Heart J* 2001; 22: 1978–90.

80. Atherton J, Thomson H, Moore T, et al. Diastolic ventricular interaction: A possible mechanism for abnormal vascular responses during volume unloading in heart failure. *Circulation* 1997; 96: 4273–9.

81. Atherton J, Moore T, Thomson H, et al. Restrictive left ventricular filling patterns are predictive of diastolic ventricular interaction in chronic heart failure. *J Am Coll Cardiol* 1998; 1: 413–18.

82. The Fragmin during Instability in Coronary Artery Disease (FRISC) study group. Low-molecular-weight heparin during instability in coronary artery disease. *Lancet* 1996; 347: 561–8.

83. Belardinelli R, Georgiou D, Scocco V, et al. Low intensity exercise training in patients with chronic heart failure. *J Am Coll Cardiol* 1995; 26: 975–82.

84. Hanumanthu S, Butler J, Chomsky D, et al. Effect of a heart failure program on hospitalization frequency and exercise tolerance. *Circulation* 1997; 96: 2842–8.

85. Coats A. Optimizing exercise training for subgroups of patients with chronic heart failure. *Eur Heart J* 1998; 19 (suppl): 029–034.

CHAPTER 6

A prospective study of an intervention specific to heart failure

Introduction

Chapter 5 described preliminary studies examining the potential beneficial effects of an essentially nurse-mediated, multidisciplinary, home-based intervention (HBI) in optimizing health outcomes in chronic heart failure. A detailed examination of the results of these studies suggested that although this type of intervention has potential benefits for most older chronically ill patients at greater risk for hospital readmission, patients with severe, chronic congestive heart failure would benefit most from its application.

However, despite strong preliminary data, the potential benefits of this intervention had not been examined in an appropriately powered, prospective study of patients with chronic heart failure that included serial measurement of functional and health-related quality of life status. Furthermore, there were limited data concerning determination of potential mechanisms of beneficial effect, which, although problematic, needed to be at least partially addressed. The preliminary study also examined the effects of a broad-based intervention that was both applicable to a heterogeneous group of chronically ill patients and involved a limited component of in-hospital counselling. For the purpose of this prospective study, therefore, it was appropriate to make the study intervention more specific to heart failure while retaining the ability to deal with issues arising from concomitant chronic disease states. Importantly, the use of a specialist cardiac care nurse with a good working knowledge of cardio-active pharmacological agents and the ability to refer patients to community-based pharmacists if required, obviated the need (and therefore incumbent costs) for a study pharmacist. Most importantly, on the basis of the need to assess the relative beneficial effects of HBI alone on subsequent outcomes and to address the needs of patients who require recurrent unplanned readmissions to hospital despite initial intervention, the following adjustments were made:

1. Deletion of the hospital-based component of the original form of this intervention.
2. Application of repeat home visits to those individuals who need frequent, recurrent unplanned readmission despite initial study intervention.

Methods

Study hypothesis

This study tested the following *null* hypothesis:

> There will be no difference in the frequency of unplanned readmissions plus out-of-hospital deaths, during a minimum of six months follow-up, among 'high-risk' patients with chronic congestive heart failure discharged to home following acute hospitalization on the basis of exposure/non-exposure to a multidisciplinary, home-based intervention incremental to usual care.

Patient cohort

As before, the study was conducted at the Queen Elizabeth Hospital, a 440-bed tertiary referral hospital servicing the north-western region of Adelaide, South Australia: an area with a disproportionate number of older and socially disadvantaged persons, and a higher prevalence of chronic illness and hospital admissions rates per capita for the region.[1] Prior to commencement of patient recruitment the study was approved by the North Western Adelaide Health Service Ethics of Human Research Committee.

Eligibility criteria

Patients admitted to the hospital under the care of the cardiology unit (and therefore the management of a cardiologist) were eligible to participate if they were aged ≥ 55 years, to be discharged to home, had chronic heart failure and a history of ≥ one admission for acute heart failure. Presence of heart failure was defined on the basis of formal demonstration (via echocardiography or radionuclide ventriculography) of impaired left ventricular systolic function (left ventricular ejection fraction [LVEF] ≤ 55%) within three months of study entry *and* persistent functional impairment indicative of New York Heart Association (NYHA) class II, III or IV status. Acute heart failure was defined on the basis of pulmonary congestion/oedema evident on chest radiography, with a clinical syndrome of acute dyspnoea at rest. Chronicity of heart failure was determined on the basis of exclusion of factors such as acute myocardial infarction (AMI) or unstable angina pectoris which might have precipitated emergence of reduced systolic function at the time of index admission and/or estimation of LVEF. However, patients admitted with acute myocardial ischaemia or infarction with previously documented heart failure were eligible for inclusion. Other exclusion criteria were presence of terminal malignancy requiring palliative care, planned corrective cardiac surgery (heart transplantation, coronary artery bypass or valve replacement) or home address outside the hospital catchment area.

Study randomization

A total of 4055 cardiology inpatients were screened over a period of 14 months starting in March 1997. Of these, 285 inpatients (7.0%) fulfilled the clinical parameters for study entry; however, 34 (11.9%) inpatients admitted from home were subsequently discharged to a long-term care facility, 21 (7.4%) refused to participate (usually on the basis of the anticipated intrusiveness of a potential home visit), 15 (5.3%) lived outside the hospital's catchment area and 10 (3.5%) were scheduled for corrective cardiac surgery (for example, coronary artery bypass or valvular replacement). Therefore, a total of 205 patients (representing 71.9% of clinically eligible patients) were recruited. Figure 6.1 represents an overview of study recruitment and design.

After signing a consent form the 205 patients were randomly allocated (via a blinded, computer-generated protocol) to either HBI or to usual care (UC). Before hospital discharge, however, five randomized patients (2.4%) died. Therefore, a total of 200 patients were subject to study follow-up (100 HBI vs 100 UC patients).

Data collection

Baseline collections

Immediately before hospital discharge patients were interviewed and their medical records reviewed to determine baseline clinical, demographic and psychosocial characteristics. Specific baseline measures included:

1. Mental acuity using the Mini-Mental State Examination.[2]
2. Functional status using both the New York Heart Association (NYHA) Classification to assess extent of dyspnoea-induced, exercise intolerance in all patients[3], the Canadian Heart Classification to assess extent of angina-induced exercise intolerance among those patients with documented ischaemic heart disease[4], and the Katz Activities of Daily Living Index to assess extent of overall functional activity.[5]
3. The extent of the concomitant disease burden using the Charlson Index of Co-morbidity, an accumulative index that adjusts for the presence of chronic congestive heart failure and myocardial infarction and that has been correlated with increased risk of death in older cohorts of hospitalized patients.[6]

Patient management

Usual care

All 200 study patients were subject to pre-existing levels of discharge planning. This included individual counselling by a cardiac rehabilitation nurse who

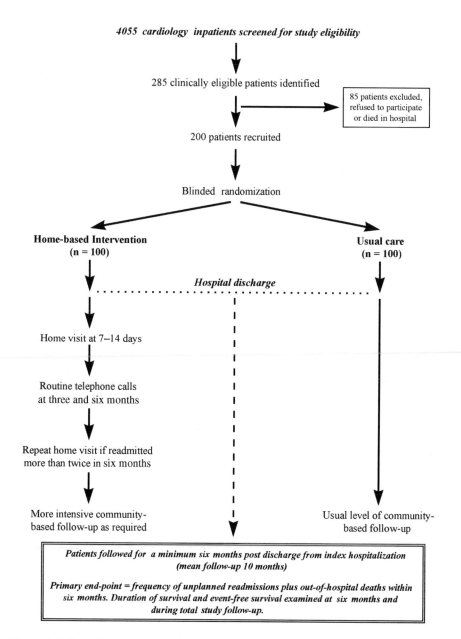

4055 cardiology inpatients screened for study eligibility

285 clinically eligible patients identified

85 patients excluded, refused to participate or died in hospital

200 patients recruited

Blinded randomization

Home-based Intervention (n = 100)

Usual care (n = 100)

Hospital discharge

Home visit at 7–14 days

Routine telephone calls at three and six months

Repeat home visit if readmitted more than twice in six months

More intensive community-based follow-up as required

Usual level of community-based follow-up

Patients followed for a minimum six months post discharge from index hospitalization (mean follow-up 10 months)

Primary end-point = frequency of unplanned readmissions plus out-of-hospital deaths within six months. Duration of survival and event-free survival examined at six months and during total study follow-up.

Figure 6.1: Overview of study recruitment and design.

reviewed the causes and consequences of heart failure and the specific treatment regimen prescribed for the patient. There was no restriction imposed on the extent and intensity of follow-up; this included both inpatient and community-based contact with dietitians, social workers, pharmacists and community nurses where appropriate. Furthermore, most patients had an appointment with their primary care physician and the cardiology outpatient clinic within two weeks of discharge. In all cases, regular outpatient-based review by the responsible cardiologist was undertaken throughout the follow-up period.

Multidisciplinary home-based intervention

Patients assigned to the HBI condition (n = 100) received the same level of care as UC patients, and also received a structured home visit by an experienced cardiac-care nurse with postgraduate qualifications, within a target period of 7–14 days after acute hospitalization. Table 6.1 outlines the principal components of this home visit in relation to the previously identified precursors of unplanned hospitalization and the remedial action that could be taken to ameliorate identified problems. Furthermore, as part of the intervention, all the patients' cardiologists and primary care physicians (if not already contacted immediately after the home

Table 6.1: Structure of home visits performed at 7–14 days post hospitalization.

Principal components of home visit	Potential problems	Actions
Review of patient's progress since hospital discharge followed by a physical examination.	Early clinical deterioration.	Urgent referral to cardiologist or primary care physician for review of current management.
Assessment of adherence to prescribed treatment.	Non-adherence to treatment regimen.	Introduce compliance device and arrange incremental pharmacist follow-up.
Assessment of understanding of disease process and purpose of treatment regimen.	Non-recognition of warning signs of impending crises.	Remedial counselling for patient and/or family. Increase frequency of community-based assessment and support.
Assessment of current level of exercise.	Peripheral muscle wasting.	Introduce simple exercise regimen (e.g. walking around the garden every day).
Assessment of current level of psychosocial support.	Poor social support systems.	Referral to social worker. Arrange more domiciliary support.
Assessment of the patient's home environment.	Danger of falling.	Arrange more appropriate bathroom and general safety equipment.

visit) received a written report of the assessments made at the visit and any remedial actions taken or recommended.

A home visit was repeated only if a patient had ≥ two unplanned readmissions within six months of the index admission. However, all surviving HBI patients were contacted by telephone at three and six months to assess their progress and arrange additional follow-up if required, and they were encouraged to contact the cardiac nurse if any subsequent problems arose and they were unsure of what action(s) to take in this regard.

Study end-points

Primary end-point

Consistent with previous studies of this type[7], the primary end-point for the study was the frequency of unplanned readmissions *plus* out-of-hospital deaths. The primary analysis of these data looked at this primary end-point during the minimum six-month follow-up of study patients, which corresponded to the duration of the study intervention.

To examine the duration of any potential benefits of the study intervention after this time, secondary analysis involved examination of this end-point and overall survival data during total patient follow-up, representing a mean of 10 ± 5 month follow-up (range 6–19 months) post index admission for the entire cohort.

Secondary end-points

A number of other pre-specified end-points were examined during the study. These included:

1. Time to first primary end-point (therefore event-free survival), unplanned readmission and death.
2. Frequency of unplanned readmissions, out-of-hospital deaths, days of unplanned readmission.
3. Cost of hospital-based health care, community-based care, functional status and health-related quality of life and knowledge of prescribed treatment within six months of the index admission.

All hospital activity, including associated costs, was monitored through the hospital's medical record and accounting departments. Records of the time and location of all deaths occurring in South Australia (via the South Australian Birth, Deaths and Marriages Registry) were used to compile mortality data. For the purpose of examining those end-points not related to hospital use and survival, patients were subjected to additional stratified randomization and were allocated (according to original study assignment) to one of the three types of specific follow-up:

1. Measurement of health-related quality of life and functional status at hospital discharge and then at three and six months thereafter using the Australian version of the SF-36[8], the Minnesota Living with Heart Failure Questionnaire[9], the Katz Activities of Daily Living Index and the NYHA and Canadian Heart (if appropriate) classifications (n = 68). Because of the relatively small numbers of patients and the large number of items comprising the SF-36, the comparison between groups was made on the basis of changes in the physical and mental health component scores derived from the instrument.
2. Estimation of total costs of community-based care, including pharmacotherapy and consultation with primary care physicians and other community-based services (n = 66).
3. Measurement of knowledge of the prescribed cardio-active agents at hospital discharge and then one and six months thereafter, using the same questionnaire for measuring medication-related knowledge as described in the previous chapter (n = 66).

Statistical analysis

Based on the results of the preliminary studies of multidisciplinary, home-based intervention among a similar cohort of patients with heart failure described in Chapter 5, we calculated that 90 patients in each group would be needed to detect a 20% variation in the composite end-point (assuming 0.5 events per UC patient during a minimum follow-up of six months with a two-side α of 0.05 and a β of 0.2).

Comparison of baseline and end-point data involved using the following:

1. χ^2 analysis (with calculation of odds ratio – OR and 95% confidence intervals where appropriate) for discrete variables.
2. Student's t test for normally distributed continuous variables.
3. Mann-Whitney test for non-normally distributed variables (this more conservative test was subsequently used for most of the major end-points).
4. Construction of Kaplan-Meier survival curves for time to first primary end-point (event-free survival) and death, followed by analysis with both the log-rank test and the Breslow test to determine any difference between groups in respect to the number and/or timing of events.

To further adjust for differences in survival and duration of study follow-up, and to reduce skewness of data, study end-points (where applicable) were calculated on the frequency of events per patient per month of study follow-up.

Examination of the interaction between treatment mode and other potential correlates of the primary end-point and overall mortality at six months post index hospitalization involved the use of a Cox Proportional Hazards Model (with entry of variables at a univariate significance level of 0.05 and backward, stepwise rejection of variables at the 0.05 level of significance).

All analyses were performed on an *intention-to-treat* basis according to study group assignment using SPSS for Windows (8.0).

Results

Baseline characteristics

Table 6.2 summarizes the clinical and demographic features of study patients according to treatment group. Analysis of baseline data suggested that the two

Table 6.2: Baseline clinical and demographic profile of study cohort.

	HBI (n = 100)	UC (n = 100)	*p* value
Demographic profile			
Male	61	59	0.772
Age in years	75.2 ± 7.1	76.0 ± 9.3	
(range)	(55–90)	(55–94)	0.495
Living alone	36	32	0.551
Primary language not English	32	32	1.000
≤ 8 years formal education	43	47	0.569
Routine home support services at discharge	43	47	
Main income – government pension	86	86	1.000
Clinical profile			
Median duration of treatment for	21.0	15.0	
chronic heart failure	(2.0–42.0)	(2.0–42.0)	0.464
Number of admissions for acute heart	2.3 ± 1.9	1.8 ± 1.1	
failure (range) *	(1–14)	(1–6)	0.033
Left ventricular ejection	36.5 ± 10.3	37.3 ± 11.4	
fraction (range)	(10–55)	(9–55)	0.624
Left ventricular ejection fraction ≤ 40%	68	60	0.239
Co-morbidity			
Ischaemic heart disease (% with known infarction)	77 (79%)	79 (67%)	0.733
Chronic airways limitation	33	38	0.459
Chronic hypertension	65	65	1.000
Atrial fibrillation	41	29	0.075
Non-insulin/insulin dependent diabetes	29:5	30:4	0.938
Mean Charlson Index of Co-morbidity score	3.0 ± 1.5	3.2 ± 1.4	0.403
Hospitalization in the six months before study follow-up			
Number of unplanned admissions (range)	1.6 ± 0.9 (1–5)	1.7 ± 1.1 (1–7)	0.308
Total days of unplanned	8.0	8.0	
hospitalization	(4.0–15.0)	(4.0–13.0)	0.986
≥ 3 unplanned admissions	16	17	0.849
Duration of index admission (days)	6.6 ± 5.8 (2–45)	6.9 ± 5.9 (2–33)	0.709

(contd)

Table 6.2: (contd).

	HBI (n = 100)	UC (n = 100)	*p* value
Index admission			
Acute pulmonary oedema	53	51	0.777
Heart rate (beats/minute)	96 ± 27	95 ± 26	0.806
Systolic blood pressure (mm Hg)	146 ± 32	147 ± 33	0.719
Diastolic blood pressure (mm Hg)	87 ± 23	87 ± 21	0.987
Sinus rhythm: atrial fibrillation	58:33	72:22	0.116
Acute myocardial ischemia	18	10	0.103
Pharmacotherapy at hospital discharge			
Number of prescribed medications	7.6 ± 2.1 (3–13)	7.6 ± 2.1 (3–14)	1.000
Diuretic	95	98	0.444
Nitrate	77	74	0.622
ACE inhibitor	75	67	0.213
Digoxin	71	60	0.102
Aspirin	69	77	0.203
Perhexiline maleate	36	33	0.655
β-adrenoceptor blocker	33	23	0.154
Warfarin	28	18	0.093
Amiodarone	18	15	0.568
Calcium antagonist	12	15	0.535
Blood profile at hospital discharge			
Sodium mmol/L	138 ± 3.5	139 ± 3.2	0.337
Potassium	4.0 ± 0.5	4.1 ± 0.6	0.356
Creatinine μmol/L *	0.138 ± 0.061	0.165 ± 0.096	0.022
Urea *	11.2 ± 5.5	13.9 ± 9.1	0.012
Albumin g/L	38.2 ± 4.3	38.8 ± 4.2	0.313
Packed cell volume	0.401 ± 0.048	0.388 ± 0.051	0.056
Platelet count	227 ± 86	227 ± 77	0.245
White cell count	9.1 ± 3.2	9.2 ± 3.1	0.854
Haemoglobin	13.4 ± 1.6	13.0 ± 1.7	0.054
Haemodynamic status at hospital discharge			
Heart rate (beats/minute)	77 ± 15	76 ± 11	0.413
Systolic blood pressure (mm Hg)	121 ± 19	124 ± 22	0.356
Diastolic blood pressure (mm Hg)	67 ± 12	66 ± 10	0.407
Sinus rhythm: atrial fibrillation	63:31	73:25	0.093
Left bundle branch block	29	19	0.098
Nutritional status at hospital discharge			
'Dry weight' (kg)	73 ± 15	70 ± 16	0.299
Cachexia	28	27	0.874

Table 6.2: (contd).

	HBI (n = 100)	UC (n = 100)	p value
Functional status at hospital discharge			
Dependent for ≥ 1 activity of daily living			
according to Katz Index	47	56	0.203
Domiciliary support	43	47	0.569
NYHA Class II : III : IV	42:46:12	48:43:9	0.628
Canadian Heart Class II : III : IV	44:24:3	41:26:3	0.977
Mini-Mental score	29.2 ± 1.8	28.8 ± 1.9	0.095

Normally distributed continuous data are presented as a mean (± one standard deviation) and skewed data are presented as a median (± interquartile range).

groups were well matched for all but three parameters (greater number of previous admissions for acute heart failure among HBI patients and higher creatinine and urea concentrations among UC patients on hospital discharge); however, on the basis of subsequent multivariate analysis, these parameters were found not to significantly influence study outcome. As expected, this was a frail and older cohort of 'high-risk' patients with chronic heart failure, most with moderate to severe systolic dysfunction and persistent symptoms despite what would be considered optimal pharmacotherapy at the time of study entry. Consistent with studies of this type, concomitant disease states including ischaemic heart disease, chronic hypertension, chronic airways limitation, diabetes, atrial fibrillation and chronic renal failure were prevalent among the study cohort.

Of the 58 patients who were not prescribed an angiotensin-converting enzyme (ACE) inhibitor at hospital discharge, 23 (40%) were unable to tolerate prior ACE inhibition because of associated renal dysfunction and a further 8 (14%) had pre-existing contraindications to ACE inhibition; all 31 of these patients were prescribed a combination of a nitrate and a diuretic plus an α receptor blocker (n = 8) and/or a β-adrenoceptor blocker (n = 9). A further 13 patients (22%) who had chronic heart failure in the absence of known ischaemic heart disease and a documented LVEF between 45% and 55% were prescribed a diuretic plus amlodipine.

Extent of multidisciplinary, home-based intervention

During the study, 88 of the 100 patients assigned to HBI (88%) received a home visit: two patients died within 48 hours of discharge and 10 patients subsequently refused the home visit despite initial consent (the last group of patients did not differ significantly from the remainder of the cohort with regard to baseline characteristics). Of the 88 initial home visits performed, 89% were within the target period of 7–14 days post discharge; the remainder were delayed because of early readmission to hospital. The median duration of these visits was 2 hours (range 1–3.5 hours).

Early clinical deterioration

Although most patients were discharged from hospital in a clinically stable state, the clinical review and physical examination undertaken by the cardiac nurse during the initial home visit showed that a large proportion of patients had signs of early clinical deterioration. In general patient heart rates were lower (77 ± 16 vs 72 ± 10 beats/min) and both systolic blood pressure (121 ± 19 vs 131 ± 19 mm Hg) and diastolic blood pressure (67 ± 12 vs 73 ± 11 mm Hg) were higher in comparison with that at hospital discharge. On an individual basis, 16 patients reported a decline in exercise intolerance to NYHA Class IV (n = 16), nine patients reported episodes of angina pectoris at rest and six patients described symptoms indicative of paroxysmal nocturnal dyspnoea. On physical examination 19 patients had basal crepitations and six patients had gross pitting oedema in the lower limbs. Overall, 35 of the 88 patients initially visited at home (40%) had one or more signs and symptoms indicative of early clinical deterioration requiring remedial action. Table 6.3 summarizes the components of 'early clinical deterioration' evident in the cohort of 90 who consented to a home visit following study randomization.

A post-hoc analysis was done to determine the independent predictors of 'non-fatal early clinical deterioration' among the 88 patients in whom it could be reliably measured (therefore excluding the 10 patients who refused a home visit) using multiple logistic regression; as before, entry of variables into the model occurred at a univariate significance level of 0.05 and backward, stepwise rejection of variables thereafter at the 0.05 level of significance. On initial univariate

Table 6.3: Profile of early clinical deterioration among the 90 patients who consented to a home visit following study randomization.

Clinical deterioration occurring within 14 days of hospital discharge	Number/proportion (95% CI) of patients (n = 90)
Sudden death at home	2/2% (0.2, 8%)
Unplanned readmission	5/6% (2, 13%)
Functional decline indicative of NYHA Class IV	16/18% (11, 27%)
New onset of angina at rest	9/10% (4, 17%)
New onset of paroxysmal nocturnal dyspnoea	6/7% (3, 14%)
New onset gross pitting oedema	6/7% (5, 18%)
One or more of the above	35/40% (30, 51%)
≥ 2 or more of the above clinical parameters	8/35 23% (10, 40%)

analysis, nine baseline parameters were found to be significantly associated with early clinical deterioration in this cohort of 88 HBI patients. These included age, LVEF, serum creatinine and urea levels at hospital discharge, co-morbidity as determined by the Charlson Index, extent of activities of daily living as determined by the Katz ADL score, presence/absence of amiodarone at hospital discharge, presence/absence of chronic airway limitation and presence/absence of diabetes (insulin or non-insulin dependent). On subsequent multivariate analysis there were only two independent determinants of non-fatal early clinical deterioration – greater age ($p = 0.008$, OR 1.1 a year) and greater comorbidity as determined by the Charlson Index ($p < 0.001$, OR 2.0 per unit score of 1).

Treatment compliance and knowledge

A combination of pill count (wherever possible) and self-report was used to assess degree of patient compliance with their prescribed treatment. On this basis, the cardiac nurse determined that 22 patients (25%) were having obvious difficulties complying with their prescribed medications, and 14 of the 34 patients who had been prescribed a strict fluid intake (41%) were non-compliant in this regard. Furthermore, 85 patients (97%) had inadequate understanding of the purpose, effect and potential adverse effects of their medications.

When asked to recall the symptoms that led to their index hospitalization, 84 patients were able to do so (85%); however, only 45 patients (51%) were able to explain (even in a simplistic way) the cause of their symptoms – for example, a build-up of fluid in their lungs causing shortness of breath.

Importantly, patients in whom early clinical deterioration was determined to be present at the initial home visit (n = 83) were significantly more likely to self-report non-compliance with their prescribed fluid restriction (nine of 15 patients) compared with those patients who seemed to be clinically stable (three of 14 patients – $p = 0.035$, OR 5.5). Similarly, patients who showed such clinical instability were also more likely to self-report difficulty in complying with their medication regimen or were found to have significantly deviated from their regimen during the pharmacological assessment (10 of 28 vs 9 of 55 – $p = 0.047$, OR 2.8).

Remedial action

On the basis of the above findings, the cardiac nurse considered it necessary to contact a patient's general practitioner during 24 of the home visits and/or the cardiology unit on 15 occasions in order to arrange either immediate review of their clinical status and therapeutic management or to simply clarify the patients' regimen for a combined total of 33 visits (38%). Moreover, the introduction of a compliance device and/or regular pharmacist review (including home visits in some cases) was arranged for 19 patients (22%). Overall, new or incremental home-support services were arranged for 23 patients (26%).

Phone follow-up

After the initial home visit 22 patients (25%) spontaneously contacted the cardiac nurse by phone in order to clarify issues of concern. In most of these cases the patients were referred to their general practitioner for remedial action. However, it was thought to be necessary for two patients to be assessed in the hospital's emergency department and they were subsequently admitted for acute, decompensated heart failure. Of the 159 routine telephone contacts made at three and six months, only six (4%) resulted in immediate referral to the patient's general practitioner.

Repeat home visits

A total of seven of 10 patients who survived ≥ two unplanned readmissions within six months and who were not discharged to long-term institutional care consented to a repeat home visit. Such home visits were shorter than initial visits (lasting between 30 and 60 minutes) and mainly involved educational reinforcement in respect to treatment compliance and early reporting of clinical deterioration. In only one instance was a patient found to have clinically deteriorated since hospital discharge; on this basis the patient's diuretic regimen was adjusted to address recurrent paroxysmal nocturnal dyspnoea.

Primary end-point

During six months follow-up, patients assigned to HBI had a total of nine out-of-hospital deaths and 68 unplanned readmissions (a total of 77 primary events) compared with 11 out-of-hospital deaths plus 118 unplanned readmissions (129 primary events) among UC patients, representing 0.2 vs 0.4 events/month of follow-up for the HBI and UC groups respectively ($p = 0.021$).

Event-free survival

In comparison with UC patients, significantly more HBI patients remained event-free at six months (51 vs 38: $p = 0.042$). Figure 6.2 shows the cumulative probability of event-free survival for the two groups during total study follow-up.

While the two probability curves suggest that the 'early' influence of HBI on the proportion of patients experiencing an event was essentially attenuated beyond six months, they also suggest that the beneficial effect of HBI on duration of event-free survival (first evident following the implementation of most initial home visits) persisted for up to nine months: the difference between groups in this respect being significant overall ($p = 0.037$).

Unplanned readmission and hospital stay

At six months HBI patients accumulated 68 vs 118 unplanned readmissions. This represented 0.14 vs 0.34 readmissions/month for the HBI and UC groups

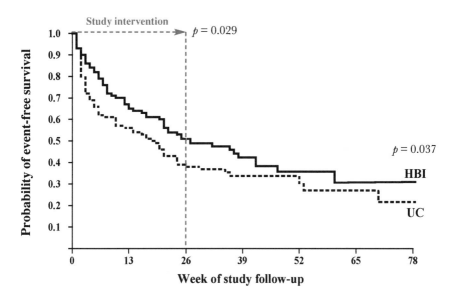

Significance levels reflect the difference between groups in respect to duration of event-free survival (Breslow/generalized Wilcoxon test).

Figure 6.2: Cumulative probability of event-free survival during study follow-up according to study assignment.

respectively ($p = 0.031$). The equivalent figures for the extended follow-up were 118 vs 156 unplanned readmissions (representing 0.15 vs 0.37 readmissions/month; $p = 0.053$). Figure 6.3 shows the accumulated total of unplanned readmissions for the two groups during study follow-up and shows that beyond six months the two groups accumulated a similar number of unplanned readmissions, essentially maintaining the early trend in favour of HBI.

Figure 6.4 also shows that the overall distribution of unplanned readmissions during six-month follow-up was significantly different for the two groups ($p = 0.042$). HBI patients were less likely to be readmitted overall and patients exposed to UC were more likely, once readmitted, to need recurrent (and costly) hospital admissions thereafter. A similar proportion of unplanned readmissions among both HBI patients and UC patients was associated with a primary diagnosis of acute heart failure, accounting for 34 (50%) vs 58 (49%) readmissions respectively. Recurrent heart failure was also the predominant reason for patients needing frequent unplanned readmissions. Not surprisingly, the HBI group required fewer days of unplanned hospitalization, accumulating a total of 460 vs 1173 days of admission (representing 0.9 vs 2.9 days/month; $p = 0.014$). Conversely, HBI patients accumulated more days of elective hospitalization, with a total of 87 vs 25

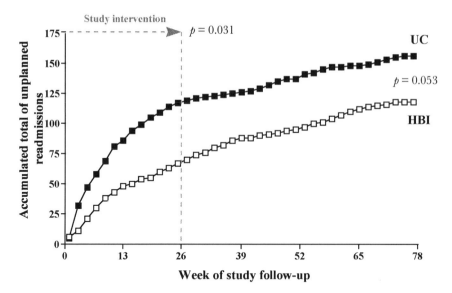

Mann-Whitney test used to compare the frequency of unplanned readmissions for the two groups.

Figure 6.3: Accumulated total of unplanned readmissions during study follow-up.

days of hospitalization ($p = 0.129$), most of which were for surgical procedures that had been previously delayed until the patient was clinically stable. During the entire study follow-up HBI patients required fewer days of unplanned hospitalization, accumulating a total of 875 vs 1476 days of admission (representing 1.1 vs 2.7 days/month; $p = 0.039$).

Mortality

At six months a total of 18 HBI patients vs 28 UC patients had died ($p = 0.098$). Figure 6.5 represents the cumulative survival curves for the two groups during the entire study follow-up. Although HBI seemed to convey an early benefit with regard to improved survival there were no statistically significant differences between groups on the basis of univariate survival analysis.

Healthcare costs

As expected, individual healthcare costs varied considerably according to the type of healthcare resource used, with HBI patients accumulating fewer hospital-based costs overall ($490,300 vs $922,600). This represented a median of $252 per HBI vs $438 per UC patient/month ($p = 0.162$): the principal difference between groups in this respect was fewer recurrent unplanned readmissions among HBI

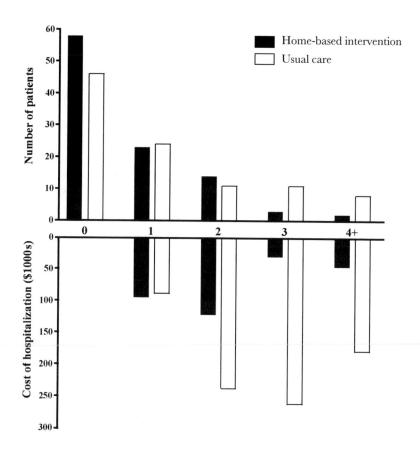

$p = 0.042$ for the comparison of the overall frequency distribution of unplanned readmissions for the two groups (χ^2 test). The costs of readmissions (above) are shown in the mirror bar graph below and are expressed in Australian dollars.

Figure 6.4: Frequency distribution of unplanned readmissions (above) and their cost (below) during six month follow-up.

patients (see Figure 6.3). Among the subset of patients for whom community-based healthcare costs were calculated ($n = 66$), expenditure was similar based on study assignment ($431 per HBI vs $438 per UC patient/month: $p = 0.91$). Alternatively, the additional cost of HBI was $350 per HBI patient.

Health-related quality of life and functional status

Table 6.4 presents the changes in health-related quality of life scores at three and six months in comparison with those collected at baseline. Consistent with

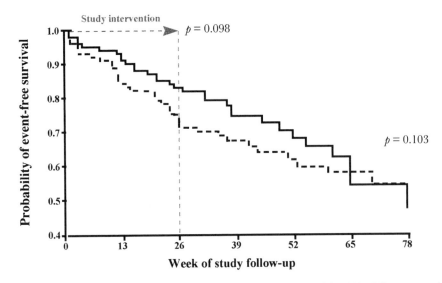

Log-rank test used to compare proportion of surviving patients with 100% follow-up at six months and mean follow-up of 10 months overall.

Figure 6.5: Cumulative probability of survival during study follow-up according to study assignment.

previous observations[10] there was a general improvement in health-related quality of life over time among surviving patients. However, although the two groups had similar baseline scores, for surviving patients at three months (62 of 68) HBI patients had significantly improved scores as measured by both the physical component score of the SF-36 and the MWLHF. Among surviving patients at six months, however, scores were similar for both groups.

Consistent with the health-related quality of life data at three and six months, patients assigned to HBI also showed better functional capacity as determined by change in NYHA functional class from baseline to three months (from 2.7 to 2.6 among HBI patients compared with 2.7 to 2.9 among UC patients), although this did not reach statistical significance ($p = 0.072$) among surviving patients. Changes in NYHA functional class from baseline to six months also favoured the HBI group (at six months the mean NYHA class of HBI patients was 2.6 compared with 2.9 among UC patients); although this difference was not statistically significant ($p = 0.105$), perhaps because of the increasing problem of Type II error.

Medication-related knowledge

Table 6.5 summarizes changes in medication-related knowledge scores at one and six months in comparison with those obtained immediately before hospital

Table 6.4: Changes in health-related quality of life scores at three and six months compared with baseline among surviving patients.

Health-related quality of life measure	HBI	UC	p value
Baseline scores	*(n = 34)*	*(n = 34)*	
Baseline MLWHF score	57 ± 21	61 ± 18	0.36
Baseline SF-36 physical health component score (%)	28 ± 11	24 ± 10	0.196
Baseline SF-36 mental health component score (%)	58 ± 22	56 ± 22	0.711
Three-month scores (comparison with baseline)	*(n = 32)*	*(n = 30)*	
δ MLWHF score	−19 (−41, 1)	−1 (−29, 10)	0.043
δ SF-36 physical health component score (%)	16 (5, 27)	3 (−8, 14)	0.014
δ SF-36 mental health component score (%)	10 (−19, 19)	6 (−9, 31)	0.483
Six-month scores (comparison with baseline)	*(n = 29)*	*(n = 24)*	
δ MLWHF score	−17 (−35, −8)	−12 (−35, −8)	0.304
δ SF-36 physical health component score (%)	17 (3, 27)	16 (3, 31)	0.526
δ SF-36 mental health component score (%)	7 (−15, 31)	19 (10, 31)	0.458

Baseline score are presented as a mean (± one SD) and subsequent scores as a median (interquartile range). Higher scores from the MLWHF (consisting of 21 questions and a score range of 0–105) indicate reduced quality of life and therefore negative changes denote improvement. Conversely, lower scores from the SF-36 (physical and mental health component scores are averaged from 5 (physical functioning, role functioning – physical, bodily pain, general health and vitality) and 3 (social functioning, role functioning – emotional and mental health) items respectively and scores range 0% to 100%) show reduced quality of life and therefore positive changes denote improvement.

Table 6.5: Changes in medication-related knowledge scores from baseline to one and six months.

Total medication-related knowledge score	HBI	UC	p value
Number of patients at baseline	*(n = 33)*	*(n = 33)*	
Mean % score at time of hospital discharge	45 ± 30	43 ± 31	0.811
Number of patients alive at one month	*(n = 31)*	*(n = 29)*	
Mean % score at three months	65 ± 28	45 ± 29	
Median δ in % score compared with baseline	11 (3, 27)	0 (−7, 7)	0.001
Number of patients alive at six months	*(n = 25)*	*(n = 21)*	
Mean % score at six months	70 ± 19	57 ± 26	
Median δ in % score compared with baseline	3 (0, 11)	1 (−3, 11)	0.290

Normally distributed continuous data are presented as a mean (± one standard deviation) and skewed data are presented as a median (interquartile range).

discharge. As expected, baseline medication scores among the subset of patients in whom this parameter was measured (n = 66) were universally poor; overall only five patients showed a good overall understanding of their prescribed cardio-active medications at the time of hospital discharge. Among surviving patients at one month post discharge, however (on average two to three weeks after the home visit), patients assigned to HBI showed a greater improvement in their understanding of their cardio-active medications in comparison with UC patients, whose scores remained consistently poor and similar to those obtained at baseline. At six months there was no longer a difference between groups in this respect, although medication-related scores among surviving HBI patients tended to be greater.

Multivariate analysis of major end-points

Based on initial univariate analysis the following variables were subject to multivariate analysis to determine independent correlates of the primary end-point (event-free survival) within six months of index hospitalization: group assignment, level of formal education, presence/absence of formal home-support services at hospital discharge, presence/absence of long-term nitrate therapy, presence/absence of long-term ACE inhibition, presence/absence of perhexiline maleate treatment, presence/absence of chronic reno-vascular disease, presence/absence of insulin/non-insulin dependent diabetes mellitus, presence/absence of sinus rhythm at hospital discharge, number of previous admissions for heart failure, extent of unplanned hospitalization in the six months before study follow-up, plasma creatinine level, haematocrit, haemoglobin level, extent of discharge pharmacotherapy, NYHA functional class, Canadian Heart functional class, Katz ADL Index score and Charlson Index score. Table 6.6 summarizes the results of the Cox Proportional Hazards Model, which revealed that the strongest independent correlates for either unplanned readmission or out-of-hospital death during this period was increased number of concomitant disease states as measured by the Charlson Index of Comorbidity, presence of formal home support services at hospital discharge, more prolonged unplanned hospitalization in the six months before study follow-up and assignment to the study intervention (which was an independent negative correlate in this respect).

As expected, unplanned readmission was the major contributor to the composite end-point. The same variables were therefore used to identify the independent correlates of unplanned readmission within six months of the index hospitalization. Table 6.7 summarizes the results of the Cox Proportional Hazards Model. Once again the Charlson Index of Co-morbidity score, extent of unplanned hospitalization in the six months before study follow-up and presence of formal home-support services at hospital discharge were strongly correlated with the need for unplanned readmission. Assignment to the study intervention was of borderline significance in this regard.

Table 6.6: Independent correlates of the primary end-point (event-free survival) during six-month follow-up according to the Cox Proportional Hazards Model.

Unplanned readmission or out-of-hospital death within six months	No (n = 89)	Yes (n = 111)	p value	Risk ratio (95% CI)
Mean (SD) Charlson Index of Co-morbidity score	2.6 ± 1.1	3.5 ± 1.5	< 0.001	1.4* (1.1, 1.8)
Routine home support services provided post hospital discharge	26 (29%)	64 (58%)	0.002	1.9 (1.5–2.3)
Mean (sd) days of unplanned hospitalization in the six months before study follow-up	8.9 ± 8.7	12.8 ± 12.5	0.009	1.02* (1.01, 1.04)
Assignment to the study intervention	51 (57%)	49 (44%)	0.031	0.66 (0.53, 0.79)

*Risk ratios were based on increments of 1 for the Charlson Index of Co-morbidity and 1 day for extent of unplanned hospitalization in the six months before study follow-up.

Table 6.7: Independent correlates of unplanned readmission during six-month follow-up according to the Cox Proportional Hazards Model.

Unplanned readmission within six months	No (n =103)	Yes (n = 97)	p value	Risk ratio (95% CI)
Mean (SD) Charlson Index of Co-morbidity score	2.5 ± 1.0	3.7 ± 1.6	< 0.001	1.5* (1.2, 1.8)
Routine home support services provided post hospital discharge	34 (33%)	56 (58%)	0.005	1.8 (1.4–2.3)
Mean (SD) days of unplanned hospitalization in the six months before study follow-up	9.0 ± 8.6	13.3 ± 13.0	0.005	1.02* (1.01, 1.04)
Assignment to the study intervention	57 (55%)	43 (44%)	0.057	0.67 (0.56, 1.0)

*Risk ratios were based on increments of 1 for the Charlson Index of Co-morbidity and 1 day for extent of unplanned hospitalization in the six months before study follow-up.

Similarly, on the basis of initial univariate analysis, the following variables were subject to multivariate analysis to determine independent correlates of death during the six month post index admission: group assignment, presence/absence of long-term nitrate therapy, presence/absence of long-term amiodarone, presence/absence of chronic reno-vascular disease, cardiac cachexia, systolic blood pressure on index admission, NYHA functional class, Katz ADL Index score, Charlson Index score, age, creatinine plasma level, Mini-Mental State Score, and LVEF.

Table 6.8 summarizes the results of the Cox Proportional Hazards Model, which showed that the strongest independent correlate for death during six-month follow-up was a longer index admission, followed by a lower LVEF, prescription of long-term nitrate therapy, a lower systolic blood pressure on index admission and assignment to the study intervention.

Discussion

Overall beneficial effects of the study intervention

The results of this randomized controlled study suggest that a relatively inexpensive, non-pharmacological intervention (HBI) augments the efficacy of pharmacotherapy in limiting readmission to hospital and death in a group of patients with severe heart failure over a period of at least six months. As such, the current data are consistent with our preliminary data presented in Chapter 5. Moreover, this is the first time that a non-pharmacological intervention of this type has been shown (as part of a prospective investigation) to both prolong event-free survival and to reduce hospital use among patients with chronic heart failure discharged from acute hospital care.

Table 6.8: Independent correlates of death during six month follow-up according to the Cox Proportional Hazards model

Death within six months of hospital discharge	No (n = 155)	Yes (n = 46)	p value	Risk ratio (95% CI)
Mean (sd) duration of index admission in days	6.0 ± 4.5	9.0 ± 8.6	< 0.001	1.07* (1.04, 1.1)
Mean (sd) left ventricular ejection fraction	38.1 ± 10.6	32.8 ± 10.9	0.011	0.97* (0.95, 0.99)
Prescribed long-term nitrate therapy at hospital discharge	110 (71%)	41 (89%)	0.015	3.7 (2.6–4.8)
Assignment to the study intervention	82 (53%)	18 (39%)	0.046	0.54 (0.0, 1.1)

*Risk ratios are based on increments of 1 day for index admission and 1% for left ventricular ejection fraction. 1 mm Hg for systolic blood pressure.

Characteristics of the study cohort

Consistent with the study cohort described in the previous chapter and with recently reported studies of hospitalized patients with heart failure[11-14], most of whom are not suitable for cardiac transplantation, this was a typically older and inherently frail cohort of patients.[15] Although the hospitalization and survival rates for the UC group in the current study are higher than those reported in recent clinical trials[15], as expected, they are comparable with the survival and hospitalization rates reported in recent studies of hospitalized patients with heart failure and specifically those observed in the epidemiological studies described in Chapter 3.[10, 11-14] For example, 54% of UC patients had an unplanned readmission within six months of the index hospitalization, and 35% had died within 12 months. As before, these figures are entirely consistent with the recent studies reported by Krumholz and colleagues (1997)[12] and Jaagosild and colleagues (1998), [10] who showed that among relatively unselected cohorts of older patients with chronic congestive heart failure, about half are readmitted within six months and one-third die within a year of an acute hospitalization. Moreover, consistent with the fact that such patients generally have a greater co-morbid burden and therefore potential for readmissions directly caused by, or complicated by, a chronic illness other than heart failure (for example, chronic pulmonary and/or reno-vascular disease)[16], in the current study 'clear-cut' admissions for heart failure accounted for only 50% of all unplanned readmissions. That extent of co-morbidity (as measured by the Charlson Index of Co-morbidity) was a major determinant of early clinical instability and unplanned readmission in this cohort of patients underscores the importance of the increased risk for poorer health outcomes among patients with multiple chronic disease states and the need for strategies that are applicable to general issues of health management rather than being entirely disease specific. Certainly, the success of HBI overall in a cohort of patients with a variety of chronic disease states, as described in Chapter 3, supports this observation.

Potential benefits of applying the study intervention

The typically poorer health outcomes among UC patients, while reflecting the limit of therapeutic impact of current pharmacological agents, represent a compelling reason for the development of adjunctive non-pharmacological treatment regimens. As discussed previously, a number of multifaceted strategies designed to address those factors associated with clinical instability and increased hospital use among patients with chronic heart failure have been evaluated in previously reported randomized[17, 18] and non-randomized studies.[19-22] Such factors include early clinical deterioration following hospital discharge[14, 18], non-adherence to treatment, [23-27] suboptimal use of healthcare services[25, 28], and the combination of poor understanding of prescribed treatment and non-recognition of clinical deterioration.[14, 29-31]

The type of HBI described in the current study was chosen for a prospective examination of its potential beneficial effects among patients with severe heart failure, on the basis of the subanalysis described in Chapter 5. As such it represents the least intensive of this type of intervention examined on a randomized basis, and, unlike those examined by Rich and Freedland[18] and Cline et al.[17], does not involve intensive (and potentially more costly) clinic-based follow-up.

Overall benefits of the study intervention

This prospective randomized study confirmed that HBI significantly reduces the frequency of unplanned readmissions, prolongs event-free survival and is associated with an overall improvement (at least in the short-term) in health-related quality of life among older patients with heart failure. Within six months of the index hospitalization HBI patients had accumulated 40% fewer unplanned readmissions and even fewer (60% less) days of unplanned hospitalization, despite the fact that more HBI patients survived the minimum six-month follow-up period. Importantly, those HBI patients subject to measurement of both heart failure-specific and general health-related quality of life had significantly better scores at three months compared with baseline. Perhaps not surprisingly, considering a previous report that the longer patients with heart failure survive an acute hospitalization the greater their quality of life[10], surviving UC patients recorded health-related quality of life scores at six months that were comparable to their HBI counterparts, suggesting that patients with relatively poorer health-related quality of life have more severe disease and are therefore more likely to die prematurely. Irrespective of the group comparison, the fact that HBI not only improved event-free survival and was associated with, at the very least, a small improvement in quality of life implies benefits not only to the healthcare system overall but to individual patients.

Is it possible to further refine the application of HBI among patients with heart failure by specifically targeting those patients who require frequent and recurrent unplanned readmissions? Post-hoc analysis of the independent determinants of frequent hospital use within the minimum six-month follow-up (defined as three or more unplanned readmissions or more than 0.5 readmissions per month of follow-up if the patient died prematurely) among UC patients (n = 100) was undertaken. According to multiple logistic regression, the only independent predictor of frequent and recurrent hospital use (n = 22) was greater number of unplanned admissions in the six months before study follow-up (1.5 vs 2.4 unplanned admissions; $p = 0.005$, adjusted OR 1.9 for increments of one unplanned admission).

Cost implications

Consistent with the results of our preliminary studies this type of intervention seems to be most cost-effective in reducing the number of patients who require

frequent and costly unplanned readmissions and thereby consume a disproportionate share of overall health expenditure (see Figure 6.3): such patients have long
been identified as the 'high-cost' users of healthcare resources.[32, 33] Whereas 18
patients assigned to UC needed more than three unplanned readmissions within
six months of the index hospitalization, only three HBI patients required the same.
Importantly, the more prolonged survival of HBI patients did not result in a
parallel increase in the number of unplanned readmissions; if this had occurred,
the early cost-benefits of HBI might have been completely attenuated in the longer
term. This suggests, therefore, that the initial savings associated with the implementation of HBI are likely to be maintained at least in the medium term.

In this context the cost of implementing HBI, and the increased community-
based healthcare services it initially engendered, were more than compensated by
the combination of savings associated with the approximate 60% reduction in
hospital stay compared with UC patients and the fact that UC patients also tended
to attract more community-based services after each hospital admission (thereby
equalizing the cost of community-based follow-up between groups over the six-
month follow-up). Consistent with previous investigations that have examined the
relative contributions of hospital versus community-based healthcare expenditure
to the overall cost of managing patients with chronic heart failure[34, 35], the
projected total of community-based healthcare costs for the UC group (based on
data from the subset of patients in whom these were estimated) was less than half
that of hospital-based costs ($440,000 vs $920,000). Because of the inherent
variability of individual costs (and therefore the skewness of data overall), the
difference between groups in respect to cost of hospital-based health care within
six months did not reach statistical significance. At the very least, however, we have
shown that the reduction in hospital use associated with HBI has the potential to
offset the cost of its implementation and is unlikely to be associated, in the medium
term at least, with greater hospital use among surviving patients.

Correlates of unplanned readmission

Of importance is the fact that the multivariate analysis (on an intention-to-treat
basis) showed that the effect of the intervention on both event-free survival and
survival alone at six months (the effective duration of the intervention and the
point in time when there was 100% follow-up) was independent of other covari-
ates. Consistent with our previous observations, extent of hospital use before study
follow-up was a reliable predictor of future hospital use, as was the presence of
routine use of home-based services which evidently acts as a good and practical
surrogate for severe functional impairment; the latter probably being more sensitive than extent of functional impairment as measured by NYHA functional class
and the more general Katz ADL Index because it also (inadvertently) takes into
consideration the patient's extent of social support and is less susceptible to the
vagaries of individual interpretation. The Charlson Index also encompasses a

number of factors and proved to be a reliable predictor of a primary event within six months. In this respect the combined score from the Charlson Index of Co-morbidity took into account the presence of multiple rather than singular factors (other than heart failure) likely to influence health outcomes (for example, the combined presence of chronic airway limitation, severe reno-vascular disease and insulin-dependent diabetes associated with end-organ damage).

Correlates of survival

Consistent with the results of the major study of patients with and without chronic cardiac disease states, and the subset analysis of patients with chronic heart failure participating in that study (both of which are described in Chapter 3), HBI was independently associated with more prolonged survival within six months. Although this does not provide definitive proof that this intervention, if applied widely, will consistently prolong survival among patients with heart failure, that a potential improvement in survival (however small it may prove to be if applied widely) is not associated with increased hospital use thereafter, and moreover seems to be associated with at least equivalent quality of life in the short term, is encouraging. Unlike the previous study, however, reduced mortality was not mediated through a reduction in out-of-hospital deaths: at six months nine HBI patients versus 11 UC patients had died without being readmitted to hospital. This was probably because non-English speaking status (the most important variable identified previously) was not significantly associated with such an event in the current study. However, since the results of previous studies have been made public, greater efforts have been made in the region to alert non-English patients about the risks of not accessing appropriate health care when needed. More consistent with previous data was the fact that mortality was independently associated with (once again) prior hospital use and reduced left ventricular systolic function. Less easy to explain is use of long-term nitrates as a negative predictor of survival. However, nitrates were prescribed (as expected) more commonly to those patients with known ischaemic heart disease and who had previously failed to tolerate ACE inhibition; both of which have been linked with poorer health outcomes in patients with heart failure.[27, 29, 36]

Prolonged beneficial effects

The more extended follow-up of those patients recruited earlier in the study suggested that the beneficial effects of HBI in respect to event-free survival persist for up to three months after the final telephone follow-up and therefore up to nine months after initial hospitalization. Although there was little difference between the proportions of patients who were event-free after 12 months, the difference between groups with respect to the accumulated total of unplanned readmissions (reaching its zenith at six months), as previously, was essentially maintained during prolonged follow-up. This is most probably a result of the combination of the repeat home visits to patients who survived more than two unplanned readmissions to the hospital within six months and the fact that the intervention was associated with a reduction in recurrent unplanned readmissions overall.

Potential mechanisms of beneficial effect

What are the essential components of this type of intervention and what are the exact mechanisms of beneficial effect? As has been discussed a number of times in this book, although it is inherently difficult to attribute direct cause and effect with multifaceted interventions of this type[18, 21, 37], the results of previous studies suggested that the relative impact of in-hospital interventions[28, 38] seem to be smaller when compared with those that incorporate a home visit and comprehensive assessment. It was postulated that the major benefit of visiting patients with heart failure in the home post acute hospitalization would be a better assessment of the patients' management of their illness(es) and a more accurate determination of their future needs. In this respect it was showed that a large proportion of patients experience early clinical deterioration likely to lead to rehospitalization without remedial intervention. Consistent with studies that have shown that this type of intervention improves treatment compliance[23] and reduces medication-related admissions, the home visit resulted in a more accurate determination of adherence to treatment and understanding of therapeutic goals, as well as implementation of longer-term strategies designed to optimize management thereafter. Not surprisingly, perhaps, patients with early clinical deterioration detected during the home visit were most likely to be found to be malcompliant with their treatment regimen and were generally older and had a greater co-morbidity. Moreover, the improvement in scores measuring knowledge of prescribed cardioactive medication at one month among the relatively small cohort of HBI patients in this study, when compared with the results presented in Chapter 5 (which showed that in-hospital counselling was relatively ineffectual in improving medication-related knowledge among a larger cohort of chronically ill patients), supports the hypothesis that educational strategies targeting older individuals in this respect are best implemented in an individual's home. In the UC group, medication-related knowledge seemed to be relatively stable at one and six months compared with baseline and remained, in most cases, suboptimal. However, the general improvement in medication-related scores among HBI patients, although promising, rarely translated into a comprehensive understanding of the prescribed medication regimen. In this context, the most important effect of home-based counselling is probably the most difficult to measure – the effect on the knowledge base of the patient's family/carers. There is only anecdotal evidence to suggest that HBI made a major impact in this regard and that this was a partial (but probably important) contributor to the overall beneficial effects of HBI.

Following an initial home visit, the combination of telephone follow-up, the occasional repeat home visit and contact with other healthcare professionals enabled the cardiac nurse to monitor the success of the initial home visit and take remedial action accordingly. However, the home visit itself seems to be the essential component of the intervention. In this respect, Figures 6.2 and 6.3 show that the two groups did not begin to diverge in respect to the primary end-point until the initial home visits were implemented and there seemed to be little to gain directly from the routine telephone contacts thereafter; although patients (and their families) almost universally appreciate the opportunity to discuss their progress and express gratitude for the interest shown in them. Although a small number of home visits were repeated as part of the current study, the results of the preliminary study (where only a single home visit was applied) support the supposition that the initial home visit has the greatest impact on subsequent health outcomes. It is possible that in other healthcare systems, arrangements for follow-up care would be less likely to occur without a structured programme thereafter (this is discussed below). However, in the context of the service provision in the north-western region of Adelaide, the cardiac nurse was able to arrange new, or increase the level of pre-existing, healthcare follow-up with a large degree of cooperation from the appropriate services (in particular general practitioners). Repeat home visits rarely provided additional insight into potential preventable reasons for patient readmission. For example, it is difficult to enforce treatment adherence once an individual has rejected previous attempts in this respect and the individual is happy to live with the consequence (however costly to the health-care system and themselves it may be). It should also be noted that, consistent with our previous experience, 10% of HBI patients refused the home visit following randomization. Although the intention-to-treat analysis showed that HBI was beneficial overall, patients who refuse additional assistance may prove to be at particular risk for poorer health outcomes: of the 10 patients who subsequently refused HBI, five died during the minimum six-month follow-up and seven experienced a primary event.

Study caveats/limitations

Despite the apparent effectiveness of HBI there are a number of issues that require comment. Although delaying the home visit to 7–14 days post-hospitalization allows potential problems to emerge (and therefore be addressed), almost 10% of HBI patients either died or were readmitted beforehand, thereby reducing its apparent efficacy. The timing of the home visit remains problematic. However, it may be possible to stratify patients in respect to immediate risk of early clinical deterioration and, on this basis, selectively apply earlier home visits. Similarly, despite the apparent longer-term effects of the current form of HBI, the intensity of routine reinforcement needed to sustain the effectiveness of initially implemented strategies remains uncertain. In the current investigation repeat home visits were applied selectively to those patients who had two or more unplanned readmissions within six months and this seemed to limit the proportion of patients requiring three or more such admissions within this time frame. However, chronic heart failure is frequently characterized by progressive clinical deterioration and regular adjustments in treatment. It may prove effective therefore to revisit patients in the home if they need an unplanned readmission beyond six months.

With advances in the pharmacological treatment of heart failure (for example, more extensive use of β-adrenoceptor blockers) it is possible that the apparent incremental benefits of applying HBI may be reduced. It is certainly possible, considering the results of the recently reported ATLAS study, which indicated that higher doses of ACE inhibitors were associated with more prolonged event-free survival and reduced hospitalization[39], that patients receiving ACE inhibition were receiving suboptimal doses. Moreover, the frequency of use of β-adrenoceptor blockers may have been higher if the study recruitment began at a later date, although there is anecdotal evidence to suggest that patients were being prescribed higher doses of ACE inhibitors and greater numbers were prescribed a β-blocker (usually carvedilol) by their treating cardiologist during the course of the study. Considering that the obvious benefits of the current pharmaco-therapeutics used in the treatment of chronic heart failure are frequently tempered by the increased risk of serious adverse effects such as deteriorating renal function secondary to ACE inhibition among such patients[40, 41], it is unlikely, in any case, that most patients enrolled in this study would be able to tolerate marked changes in their treatment regimen and/or derive the type of clinical benefits reported in recent clinical trials. Moreover, as discussed and shown in the previous chapter, greater number of medications and associated adjustments in dosage increase the probability for both non-adherence and development of adverse effects. Importantly, considering the association between both non-specialist management and inappropriate pharmacotherapy with poorer health outcomes[11, 41–45], all study patients were being managed by a cardiologist and receiving treatment appropriate to current guidelines at the time of study recruitment.[46]

Are the results of this study applicable to other countries and healthcare systems? Although these issues will be discussed in more detail in the next chapter (a formal comparison of this cohort with one in the UK), it is worth noting that this study was performed at a single institution. As discussed earlier, the results of this study are both consistent with the preliminary studies described in Chapter 5 and those studies emanating from the USA[18–21] and Europe.[17, 47] Moreover, preventable hospital readmissions are a phenomenon common to nearly all developed countries[25] and this study provides further evidence that interventions that can accurately identify and address the preventable factors that lead to unplanned hospitalization will prove to be cost-effective if implemented widely and targeted towards higher-risk individuals. It is almost inevitable that such an intervention will need to be modified to meet the gaps in service provision inherent to each particular healthcare system (for example, incorporating nurse-led heart failure clinics to ensure planned strategies are implemented following a home visit).[48, 49]

Although the exact mechanism(s) of beneficial effect of exercise programmes for patients with heart failure are yet to be elucidated, it is possible that HBI could prove to have synergistic effects when combined with proven programmes of this type[50–52]; especially among relatively stable patients who have less severe functional impairment.[53] Because it has been suggested that even low-intensity exercise regimens can improve exercise capacity[54], many HBI patients were encouraged to take a short walk every day as part of the intervention. However, considering the fact that this was an inherently older and frail cohort of patients with clinically unstable heart failure, it is difficult to determine what effect this component of the intervention had on subsequent outcomes, especially as many of the study patients had a concomitant illness that limited exercise (for example, rheumatoid arthritis and severe chronic airways limitation) and therefore found it difficult to mobilize at all. Such patients may derive incremental benefits from the introduction of a single limb training regimen.[55] Despite the practical difficulties inherent to the application of an exercise regimen among this type of patient cohort, the increasing evidence that an exercise regimen will improve a patient's health status, regardless of their clinical profile, suggests that a more formal exercise component could be introduced into this type of intervention, especially as HBI seems to optimize the effect of pre-existing pharmacotherapy and lead to greater clinical stability.

Finally, it is also inevitable that HBI patients received more considerate and comprehensive care because they were allocated to active intervention (this would be most obvious to the treating cardiologist and general practitioner following receipt of the cardiac nurse's report as a result of the initial home visit). Although this is a non-specific effect that is obviously difficult to control, it is unlikely that the inherent bias of being an intervention patient would account entirely for the magnitude of beneficial effect associated with HBI. Furthermore, the provision of more comprehensive and considerate care is one of the major objectives of this and other types of multidisciplinary intervention and any 'placebo' effect of HBI is likely to be sustained in the normal clinical setting.

Summary

In establishing a strong case for a true cause and effect relationship between HBI and reduced unplanned readmissions and prolonged event-free survival among older patients with chronic congestive heart failure, it was shown in this prospective randomized controlled study that:

- The initial effect of HBI on event-free survival (and possibly survival alone) first appears at the approximate time of the initial home visit, suggesting a temporal relationship between the two. Moreover, although the effect of the intervention on frequency of unplanned readmissions seems to be sustained for the medium term, importantly, its effect on event-free survival seems to diminish over the same period.

- The relationship between HBI and prolonged event-free survival (and survival alone) is both significant and independent of other influencing variables as determined by multivariate analysis.
- In the current study the results of the study described in Chapter 5 were essentially replicated. Furthermore, these results are entirely consistent with the current literature – including those studies due to be published in the next year or so (see Chapter 7).

Therefore, despite a number of limitations, we have demonstrated (probably for the first time) that a relatively unique and inexpensive non-pharmacological intervention of this type has the potential to significantly improve health outcomes among older individuals with chronic heart failure over the medium term through both reduced unplanned readmission and (possibly) prolonged survival. As such, HBI seems to improve patient care and subsequent health outcomes while reducing overall healthcare costs. It therefore represents an attractive adjunct to the current management of chronic heart failure and may prove to be useful in the management of other chronic cardiac disease states associated with frequent hospital use (for example, atrial fibrillation[56]).

References

1. Glover J, Sharnd M, Foster C, et al. *A Social Health Atlas of South Australia* (2nd edition). Adelaide: Policy and Budget Division, South Australian Health Commission, 1996.
2. Folstein M, Folstein S, McHugh P. Mini-Mental State. A practical method for grading the cognitive state of patients for the clinician. *J Psychiatric Res* 1975; 12: 189–98.
3. The New York Heart Association. *Diseases of the Heart and Blood Vessels; Nomenclature and Criteria for Diagnosis* (6th edition). Boston, MA: Little, Brown, 1964.
4. Campeau L. Grading of angina pectoris. *Circulation* 1975; 54: 522.
5. Katz S, Ford A, Moskowitz R, et al. The index of ADL: A standardized measure of biological and pyschosocial function. *JAMA* 1963; 185: 914–19.
6. Charlson ME, Pompei P, Ales KL, et al. A new method of classifying prognostic co-morbidity in longitudinal studies: Development and validation. *J Chron Dis* 1987; 40: 373–83.
7. Rich MW, Beckham V, Wittenberg C, et al. A multidisciplinary intervention to prevent the readmission of elderly patients with congestive heart failure. *New Engl J Med* 1995; 333: 1190–5.
8. Ware J, Sherbourne C. The MOS 36-item short-form health survey (SF-36): Conceptual framework and item selection. *Med Care* 1992; 30: 473–83.
9. Rector TS, Kubo SH, Cohn JN. Validity of the Minnesota Living with Heart Failure Questionnaire as a measure of therapeutic response to Enalapril or placebo. *Am J Cardiol* 1993; 71: 1106-07.

10. Jaagosild P, Dawson N, Thomas C, et al. Outcomes of acute exacerbation of severe congestive heart failure. *Arch Intern Med* 1998; 158: 1081–9.

11. Reis SE, Holubkov R, Edmundowicz D et al. Treatment of patients admitted to hospital with congestive heart failure: Specialty-related disparities in practice patterns and outcomes. *J Am Coll Cardiol* 1997; 30: 733–8.

12. Krumholz HM, Parent EM, Tu N, et al. Readmission after hospitalisation for congestive heart failure among medicare beneficiaries. *Arch Intern Med* 1997; 157: 99–104.

13. Burns RB, McCarthy EP, Moskowitz MA, et al. Outcomes for older men and women with congestive heart failure. *J Am Geriatr Soc* 1997; 45: 276–80.

14. Lowe J, Candlish P, Henry D, et al. Management and outcomes of congestive heart failure: A prospective study of hospitalised patients. *MJA* 1998; 168: 115–18.

15. Petrie M, Berry C, Stewart S, et al. Older hearts in failure. *Eur Heart J* (in press).

16. Brown A, Cleland J. Influence of concomitant disease on patterns of hospitalization in patients with heart failure discharged from Scottish hospitals in 1995. *Eur Heart J* 1998; 19: 1063–9.

17. Cline C, Israelsson B, Willenheimer R, et al. A cost effective management programme for heart failure reduces hospitalisation. *Heart* 1998; 80: 442–6.

18. Rich MW, Freedland KE. Effect of DRG's on three-month readmission rate of geriatric patients with congestive heart failure. *Am J Publ Hlth* 1988; 78: 680–4.

19. West J, Miller N, Parker K, et al. A comprehensive management system for heart failure improves clinical outcomes and reduces medical resource utilization. *Am J Cardiol* 1997; 79: 58–63.

20. Kornowski R, Zeeli D, Averbuch M, et al. Intensive home-care surveillance prevents hospitalization and improves morbidity rates among elderly patients with severe congestive heart failure. *Am Heart J* 1995; 129: 162–6.

21. Fonarow GC, Stevenson LW, Walden JA, et al. Impact of a comprehensive heart failure management program on hospital readmissions and functional status of patients with advanced heart failure. *J Am Coll Cardiol* 1997; 30: 725–32.

22. Hanumanthu S, Butler J, Chomsky D, et al. Effect of a heart failure program on hospitalization frequency and exercise tolerance. *Circulation* 1997; 96: 2842–8.

23. Rich MW, Gray DB, Beckham V, et al. Effect of a multi-disciplinary intervention on medication compliance in elderly patients with congestive heart failure. *Am J Med* 1996; 101: 270–6.

24. Stewart S, Pearson S. Uncovering a multitude of sins: Medication management in the home post acute hospitalisation among the chronically ill. *Austr NZ J Med* 1999; 29: 220–7.

25. Michalsen A, König G, Thimme W. Preventable causative factors leading to hospital admission with decompensated heart failure. *Heart* 1998; 80: 437–41.

26. Gooding J, Jette AM. Hospital readmissions among the elderly. *J Am Geriatr Soc* 1985; 33: 595–601.

27. Vinson JM, Rich MW, Sperry JC, et al. Early readmission of elderly patients with congestive heart failure. *J Am Geriatr Soc* 1990; 38: 1290–5.

28. Naylor M, Brooten D, Jones R, et al. Comprehensive discharge planning for the hospitalized elderly. *Ann Intern Med* 1994; 120: 999–1006.

29. Blyth F, Lazarus R, Ross D, et al. Burden and outcomes of hospitalisation for congestive heart failure. *MJA* 1997; 167: 67–70.

30. Furlong S. Do programmes of medicine self-administration enhance patient knowledge, compliance and satisfaction? *J Adv Nurs* 1996; 23: 1254–62.

31. Veggeland T, Fagerheim KU, Ritland T, et al. Do patients know enough about their medication? A questionnaire among cardiac patients discharged from 5 Norwegian hospitals. *Tidsskrift for Den Norske Laegeforening* 1993; 113: 3013–16.

32. Anderson GF, Steinberg EP. Hospital readmissions in the Medicare population. *N Engl J Med* 1984; 311: 1349–53.

33. Zook CJ, Moore FD. High-cost users of medical care. *N Engl J Med* 1980; 302: 996–1002.

34. McMurray J, Hart W, Rhodes G. An evaluation of the cost of heart failure to the National Health Service in the UK. *Br J Med Econ* 1993; 6: 99–110.

35. McMurray JJV, Stewart S. Epidemiology, aetiology and prognosis of heart failure. *Heart* 2000; 83: 596–602.

36. Franciosa JA, Wilen M, Ziesche S, et al. Survival in men with severe chronic left ventricular failure due to either coronary heart disease or idiopathic dilated cardiomyopathy. *Am J Cardiol* 1983; 51: 831–6.

37. Alessi CA, Stuck AE, Aronow HU, et al. The process of care in preventive in-home comprehensive geriatric assessment. *J Am Geriatr Soc* 1997; 45: 1044–50

38. Fitzgerald JF, Smith DM, Martin DK, et al. A case manager intervention to reduce readmissions. *Arch Intern Med* 1994; 154: 1721–9.

39. Packer M, Poole-Wilson P, Armstrong P, et al. Comparative effects of low-dose versus high-dose lisinopril on survival and major events in chronic heart failure: The Assessment of Treatment with Lisinopril and Survival study (ATLAS). *Eur Heart J* 1998; 19(suppl): 142.

40. MacDowall P, Kaira P, O'Donoghue D, et al. Risk of morbidity from renovascular disease in elderly patients with congestive cardiac failure. *Lancet* 1998; 352: 13–16.

41. Pearson TA, Peters TD. The treatment gap in coronary artery disease and heart failure: Community standards and the post-discharge patient. *Am J Cardiol* 1997; 80(suppl): 45H–52H.

42. McDermott M, Lee P, Mehta S, et al. Patterns of angiotensin-converting enzyme inhibitor prescriptions, educational interventions, and outcomes among hospitalized patients with heart failure. *Clin Cardiol* 1998; 21: 261–8.

43. Luzier A, Forrest A, Adelman M, et al. Impact of angiotensin-converting enzyme inhibitor underdosing on rehospitalization rates in congestive heart failure. *Am J Cardiol* 1998; 82: 465–9.

44. Stafford RS, Saglam D, Blumenthal D. National patterns of angiotensin-converting enzyme inhibitor use in congestive heart failure. *Arch Intern Med* 1997; 157: 2460–4.

45. Edep ME, Shah NB, Tateo IM, et al. Difference between primary care physicians and cardiologists in management of congestive heart failure: Relation to practice guidelines. *J Am Coll Cardiol* 1997; 30: 518–26.

46. Williams J, Bristow M, Fowler M, et al. Guidelines for the evaluation and management of heart failure. Report of the American College of Cardiology/American Heart Association Task Force on Practice Guidelines (Committee on Evaluation and Management of Heart Failure). *J Am Coll Cardiol* 1995; 26: 1376–98.

47. Jaarsma T, Halfens R, Huijer Abu-Saad H, et al. Effects of education and support on self-care and resource utilization in patients with heart failure. *Eur Heart J* 1999; 20: 673–82.

48. Erhardt L, Cline C. Heart failure clinics: A possible means of improving care (editorial). *Heart* 1998; 80: 428–9.

49. Strömberg A. Heart failure clinics (editorial). *Heart* 1998; 80: 426–7.

50. Conn E, Williams R, Wallace A. Exercise responses before and after physical conditioning in patients with severely depressed left ventricular dysfunction. *Am J Cardiol* 1982; 49: 296–300.

51. Letac B, Cribier A, Desplanches J. A study of left ventricular function in coronary patients before and after physical training. *Circulation* 1977; 56: 375–8.

52. Williams R. Exercise training of patients with ventricular dysfunction and heart failure. *Cardiovasc Clin* 1985; 15: 218–31.

53. Coats A. Optimizing exercise training for subgroups of patients with chronic heart failure. *Eur Heart J* 1998; 19 (suppl): O29–O34.

54. Belardinelli R, Georgiou D, Scocco V, et al. Low intensity exercise training in patients with chronic heart failure. *J Am Coll Cardiol* 1995; 26: 975–82.

55. Koch M, Douard H, Broutset J. The benefit of graded physical exercise in chronic heart failure. *Chest* 1992; 101 (suppl): 231S–5S.

56. Stewart S, MacIntyre K, McCleod MC, et al. Trends in hospital activity, morbidity and case fatality related to atrial fibrillation in Scotland, 1986–1996. *Eur Heart J* 2001; 22: 693–701.

CHAPTER 7

Nurse-led interventions in chronic heart failure: The way forward?

Introduction

In the first few chapters of this book it was established that heart failure is a significant burden on the both the healthcare system and the individual. Despite some preliminary evidence that this modern-day epidemic may be starting to reach its peak and that recent treatment strategies may be having some influence in respect to improving prognosis, there is much to be done to improve health outcomes in chronic heart failure. The last two chapters have described a remarkably successful intervention that has the potential to significantly improve outcomes related to heart failure. Before any appraisal of the merits of nurse-led interventions in chronic heart failure is made, however, it is vitally important to place such research in the context of the global effort to optimize management of heart failure – hence this chapter, which critically reviews the literature to date and presents some evidence to suggest that it is possible for international cross-fertilization in respect to applying strategies of this type.

The evidence supporting the widespread introduction of specialist nurse-led strategies in the post discharge management of chronic heart failure

Randomized controlled studies

To date (please refer to the section on 'new' studies, pp. 164–5), there have been eight randomized controlled studies that have been appropriately powered and have had complete follow-up of non-pharmacological interventions designed to prevent readmission in patients with chronic heart failure discharged from acute hospital care.

These randomized controlled studies can be categorized according to the effect of the study intervention on subsequent healthcare use relative to usual care.

One negative trial

Perhaps unsurprisingly, considering the inherent publication bias towards the reporting of positive studies, there is only one reported negative study of this type in the literature. Weinberger and colleagues described a study in which 1396 veterans (all men) hospitalized with chronic obstructive pulmonary disease, diabetes or heart failure were randomized to either usual care or to increased access to primary care nurses and physicians.[1] Although study patients received this extra care, they had a greater number of readmissions to hospital, but were more satisfied with their medical care relative to usual care during six-month follow-up. It was postulated at the time that the increased use of health care seen in the study group resulted from a combination of greater vigilance in detecting problems and the ability of those detecting such problems (the physicians) to admit patients – thereby lowering admission thresholds.[2] This so-called 'clinical cascade' effect represents an important caveat when considering the potential impact of this type of intervention. As such, although some notable commentators in this field would consider this particular study and its results as having little relevance to more comprehensive, heart failure-specific programmes[3], I would argue to the contrary. Although increased nursing contact with patients is likely to result in more clinical problems being detected, there is also the potential for increased hospitalization rates if a specialist nurse is empowered to directly admit patients to hospital.

Trials with equivocal results

In 1994 Naylor and colleagues described a controlled study of a comprehensive discharge planning protocol implemented by advanced practice nurses. Completed in 1992, this study showed short-term, but not sustained, reductions in readmissions and decreased costs of care for older hospitalized patients with a number of medical cardiac conditions (including heart failure) who were managed according to this protocol.[4] More recently, this group of researchers has examined the effects of this protocol plus a component of home-based follow-up (a series of home visits by advanced practice nurses). They reported that the intervention was associated with fewer hospital readmissions and days of associated hospitalization within 24 weeks, although only a small proportion of patients had chronic heart failure and there was a significant amount of loss to follow-up (about 30%).[5]

More recently, Jaarsma and colleagues (1999) examined the effects of a heart failure-specific, home-based educational programme undertaken by a nurse specialist in heart failure. This study was specifically undertaken to determine whether a single-type intervention designed to increase chronic heart failure patients' self-care behaviour was sufficiently effective enough to reduce hospital readmissions by a significant margin. Despite sufficient sample size, this study showed that while education alone had the potential to reduce hospital readmissions overall, cost-effective thresholds were not reached. For example, during nine-month follow-up 37% of intervention patients (n = 84) compared with 50% of usual care patients (n = 95) were readmitted to hospital ($p = 0.06$). Patients exposed to the study intervention also tended to have fewer cardiac-related days of readmission than usual care patients (427 vs 681 days; $p = 0.096$).[6]

Although the studies described above may seem to provide inconclusive proof concerning the relative merits of additional inpatient discharge planning and post-discharge home-based education, they are clearly important for a number of reasons. First, they provide a clear indication that they are inherently valuable strategies – even if not associated with a clinically significant reduction in health-care use. Second, when combined with other types of strategies, they have the potential to be cost-effective in reducing hospital readmissions.

Positive trials

In the first properly powered and conducted study of its type, Rich and colleagues reported that a nurse-led, multidisciplinary intervention (which involved a compon-ent of home visits) had beneficial effects on rates of hospital readmission, quality of life and cost of care within 90 days of discharge among 'high-risk' patients with chronic heart failure. The intervention consisted of comprehensive education of the patient and family, a prescribed diet, social service consultation and planning for an early discharge, optimization of pharmacotherapy, and intensive home and clinic-based follow-up with frequent telephone contact. On this basis, the inter-vention was successful and seemed to slow the typical cycle of recurrent hospital-ization in this type of patient cohort. At 90 days, survival without readmission was achieved in 91 of 142 (64%) intervention patients compared with 75 of 140 (54%) control patients ($p = 0.09$). There were 94 vs 53 readmissions in the control and intervention groups respectively ($p = 0.02$). Of the total readmissions 78 (53%) were for heart failure and there was a disproportionate reduction (56%) of these types of readmissions in the intervention group (24 vs 54; $p = 0.04$). Importantly, fewer patients in the intervention group had more than one readmission (9 vs 23; $p = 0.01$). These results were associated with significantly better quality of life and reduced health costs among intervention patients.[7]

In 1998, Cline and colleagues also reported the benefits of a clinic-based follow-up of a lower-risk cohort of patients with chronic heart failure.[8] A total of 206 older patients hospitalized with heart failure were randomized to the study intervention or to usual care. The special intervention included an education programme for patients and their families, concentrating on treatment. Guidelines for adjusting treatment in response to sodium and water over-load and fluid deple-tion was also provided. This programme was carried out over two 30-minute visits to the patient in hospital and a one-hour home visit to the patient and family two weeks after discharge. Frequent and easily accessible patient-initiated follow-up was provided as a nurse-run, hospital-based clinic and telephone contact. During

12-month follow-up, time to first readmission was a third longer in the intervention group (106 vs 141 days; $p < 0.05$). The intervention was also associated with a strong trend towards fewer hospital admissions, fewer days of hospitalization and lower cost of care during study follow-up; in comparison with those of Rich and colleagues.[7] It is likely that Type II error prevented the intervention from being shown to be significantly better in this regard. The results of this study therefore tend to reinforce the need to select a higher-risk subset of patients in order to target intervention in a cost-efficient manner.

As discussed in Chapters 5 and 6, following post-hoc analyses of a large-scale randomized controlled study of chronically ill patients with a mixture of cardiac and non-cardiac disease states[9], which showed that a nurse-led, multidisciplinary, home-based intervention was most effective in patients with chronic heart failure[10, 11], we prospectively examined a more heart failure-specific form of a nurse-led, home-based intervention.[12] Patients with chronic heart failure discharged home post acute hospitalization were randomized to usual care (n = 100) or to multidisciplinary, home-based intervention (n = 100). The intervention primarily consisted of a home visit at 7–14 days post discharge by a cardiac nurse to identify and address issues likely to result in unplanned hospitalization. The primary end-point for the study was frequency of unplanned readmission plus out-of-hospital death within six months. During six-month follow-up the primary end-point occurred more frequently in the usual care group (129 vs 77 primary events; $p = 0.02$). More intervention patients remained event-free (38 vs 51; $p = 0.04$). Overall, there were fewer unplanned readmissions (68 vs 118; $p = 0.03$) and associated days of hospitalization (460 vs 1173; $p = 0.02$) among patients assigned to the study intervention. Consequently, hospital-based costs for the intervention group tended to be lower than those for usual care (A\$490,300 vs \$922,600; $p = 0.16$). The mean cost of the intervention was A\$350 a patient, whereas other community-based costs were similar for both groups. The frequency distribution of unplanned readmissions was significantly different for the two groups ($p = 0.04$) with fewer patients in the intervention group (5 vs 19) requiring ≥ 3 readmissions. In a subgroup of 68 patients, heart failure specific ($p = 0.04$) and general quality of life scores ($p = 0.01$) at three months were most improved among those assigned to multidisciplinary, home-based intervention. Furthermore, assignment to the study intervention was an independent predictor of survival at six months (adjusted relative risk 0.54; $p = 0.046$).[12]

New randomized studies

A number of new, appropriately powered and designed randomized studies examining the benefits of this type of intervention have been completed in recent years and will appear in the literature in the near future. For example, Blue and colleagues have also shown the benefits of a nurse-led, home-based intervention in Glasgow, Scotland, in a patient cohort similar to those described in the study described in Chapter 6 (see below).[13, 14] Similarly, in the US, Moser and colleagues have shown that a home-based intervention is effective in patients in Ohio with chronic heart failure associated with both systolic and diastolic dysfunction[15], and Krumholz and colleagues[16] and Riegel and colleagues[17] are due to report on studies examining some residual issues concerning this type of intervention. All of these studies support the use of a home-based approach. A large trial due to be completed in the near future also merits a mention as it is being undertaken by De Busk and colleagues – the same investigators responsible for the MULTI-FIT programme. Although these studies have predominantly concentrated on home-based strategies, there are still studies examining the effect of clinic-based strategies. The most notable of these is a study describing the effects of the Auckland Heart Failure Management programme by Doughty and colleagues in New Zealand.[18] As with the Cline study, which examined a similar strategy in Sweden[8], despite some benefits incremental to usual care, its results suggest that a clinic-based approach is probably inferior to one that incorporates a home-based intervention but still provides enough evidence that a combined home- and clinic-based approach may be effective (we are currently undertaking a randomized trial of this combined approach in York, UK).

Non-randomized studies

The results of the randomized studies described above are broadly consistent with those of non-randomized studies of similar strategies targeting older, hospitalized patients with heart failure. For example, Kornowski and colleagues (1995) reported that an intensive home-based intervention by physicians was associated with reduced hospitalization rates and improved quality of life in such patients (n = 42).[19] Similarly, West and colleagues (1997) have reported that an intensive physician-supervised, nurse-mediated, home-based system for heart failure management (the MULTI-FIT programme) is associated with improved functional status and exercise capacity and reduced hospitalization rates among both previously hospitalized and clinic-managed patients with heart failure (n = 51).[20] Fonarow and colleagues (1997) have also reported favourable effects associated with a comprehensive management programme targeting younger patients with heart failure awaiting heart transplantation.[21] More recently, Shah and colleagues have reported a preliminary study examining a nurse-led monitoring programme incorporating a strategy to facilitate patient self-monitoring of their heart failure status in addition to weekly reminder calls by nurses. In a small cohort of both older and middle-aged patients with heart failure (n = 27) this strategy seemed to reduce subsequent hospitalizations.[22]

Which type of specialist nurse-led intervention is best?

Based on the literature to date, in addition to those studies already reported at major scientific meetings, it would seem that those interventions that involve a component of specialist nurse-led, home-based follow-up are more effective than those that incorporate clinic-based follow-up. Similarly, a clinic-based approach seems to be more effective than strategies confined to the period of acute hospitalization (for example, incremental discharge planning).

The results of those studies examining the effect of home-based intervention (as described in Chapter 6) suggest that such programmes have the potential to prolong event-free survival, to reduce the number of readmissions within a year of index hospitalization by about 50% and to prolong survival without adversely affecting quality of life. However, simply visiting patients at home and counselling them is obviously not enough[6] and a multidisciplinary approach is more effective.

These conclusions are largely based on randomized controlled studies. A number of historical control studies undertaken in the US suggest that a clinic-based approach might be more beneficial than home-based intervention. However, it should be noted that such studies should be interpreted with caution as they have an inherent bias in favour of the intervention by counting the qualifying event as an end-point during the historical control period.

If patients were not willing to be managed by a specialist nurse using a home-based approach then they would certainly benefit from being managed through a specialist nurse-led outpatient clinic. Moreover, excepting the study performed by Rich and colleagues[7], which limited follow-up to three months, there is a paucity of studies examining the potential value of the combination of specialist nurse-led home and clinic-based follow-up. This type of approach may prove to be the most effective of all. Furthermore, the optimal timing and frequency of interventions that have already been proven to be effective are yet to be firmly established.

Residual issues

Although specialist nurse-led interventions have been shown to be effective in improving health outcomes in chronic heart failure, this is still an evolving field of health care. As such, there are a number of important issues that remain unresolved:

- Is it possible to extrapolate results from one country to another, considering that, unlike the large-scale clinical trials, nurse-mediated interventions tend to involve a smaller number of patients at a local level?
- What is the future role of this type of intervention given the evolving armoury of pharmacological agents?
- What are the minimal qualifications for a specialist nurse in heart failure for he or she to be effective?

- Who should oversee the role and actions of the specialist nurse and how independent should they become?
- What is the optimal method for integrating a specialist nurse service into the pre-existing healthcare structure?
- How do you measure and maintain the quality of this type of intervention?
- Most importantly, who should fund this type of intervention?

Certainly, translating research into practice puts additional pressure on the architects of such interventions to apply only the essential components of their intervention. Fortunately, there are some good models on which services can be established – for example, the Glasgow Heart Failure Nurse Liaison Service in Scotland, which is based on both the Scottish and Australian experience of home-based intervention.[13, 14, 23] Indeed, the parallel studies done in Scotland and Australia have permitted us to examine at least one of the issues raised above – is it possible to extrapolate data from one country to another?

Poles apart, but are they the same? A comparative study of Australian and Scottish patients with chronic heart failure[24]

Rationale

Recent reports from large clinical trials and registries have shown considerable international variation in the use of particular medications for chronic heart failure.[25–27] Prior to this study, however, there is a paucity of data to make international comparisons in respect to patients with chronic heart failure not participating in clinical trials. We do not know, for example, whether the reported differences in treatment affect outcome or whether different healthcare systems have an influence on hospitalization rates, independently of the syndrome of heart failure itself. Furthermore, the large clinical trials, to date, have recruited subjects unrepresentative of patients with heart failure in general. Elderly people and women have, in particular, been excluded.[28]

As discussed above, two trials of specialist nurse intervention in chronic heart failure conducted in Adelaide, Australia[5], and Glasgow, Scotland, have been recently completed.[14] The design of these studies was very similar, thus allowing comparison between the baseline characteristics and subsequent health outcomes of participating patients. We have taken the opportunity offered by these recent developments to, for the first time, compare the characteristics and outcomes in hospitalized patients with heart failure in two different countries.

Methods

Patient cohorts

Both controlled studies of specialist nurse intervention in heart failure commenced recruitment in their respective countries in March 1997 and enrolled patients until the latter half of 1999. The relevant institution's ethics committee approved each study and all study patients consented to participate. As such, both studies conformed to the principles outlined in the Declaration of Helsinki. As described in Chapter 6, in Australia, a total of 205 patients were recruited from the north-west region of Adelaide, a metropolitan area with a disproportionate number of elderly and socially disadvantaged persons and higher admission rates per capita for the region.[8] All patients were admitted to the Queen Elizabeth Hospital, a tertiary referral hospital servicing the area. A total of 200 patients were subsequently discharged alive and were randomized to either usual care (n = 100) or the study intervention (n = 100). Similarly, 165 Scottish patients were recruited from the north-west sector of the city of Glasgow, which is also a metropolitan region with a disproportionate number of elderly and socially disadvantaged persons and higher admission rates compared with the overall population.[9] All patients were admitted to the Western Infirmary, a tertiary referral hospital servicing the area. A total of 158 patients were discharged alive and were randomized to either usual care (n = 75) or the study intervention (n = 83).

Patient characteristics

Both studies required patients to have a diagnosis of chronic heart failure with documented left ventricular systolic dysfunction and an associated hospitalization where heart failure was the primary cause. In the Scottish study, the index admission represented the qualifying hospitalization related to heart failure. In the Australian study the qualifying hospitalization may have occurred previously. In both studies patients were discharged home and resided in the hospitals' catchment areas.

Both studies had minimal exclusion criteria. Neither had upper age limits (although the study in Adelaide required patients to be aged ≥ 55 years) nor excluded patients on the basis of co-morbidity. However, patients were excluded on the basis of reversible ischaemia precipitating their qualifying hospitalization, valvular heart disease amenable to surgical correction, intended cardiac transplantation and presence of non-cardiac, terminal disease.

There were some differences between the two cohorts. Patients recruited into the Scottish study were admitted to hospital under the care of a general physician whereas all patients recruited in Australia were admitted under the care of a cardiologist. Moreover, in the Scottish study left ventricular systolic dysfunction was defined on a semi-quantitative scoring system of the patient's echocardiogram with a requirement for at least 'mild' dysfunction to be evident. In Australia a similar, but more quantitative, criterion of a documented LVEF of ≤ 55% was required for study entry.

Usual care

Neither study limited extent of in-hospital or post-discharge care. In Australia, patients were reviewed at regular intervals by both their general practitioner and cardiologist. In Scotland, patients were followed up by their general practitioner and cardiologist or general physician.

Study follow-up

All Australian and Scottish patients in these two studies were followed up for at least three months post discharge. Data collected from both studies permitted estimation of event-free survival (unplanned readmission or out-of-hospital death), number and frequency of unplanned readmissions, associated hospital stay and survival overall.

Statistical analysis

Univariate comparison of the baseline characteristics of the two cohorts (a total of 375 patients) and subsequent health outcomes among patients assigned to 'usual care' (a total of 175 patients) involved using the following: χ_2 analysis (with calculation of odds ratio [OR] and 95% confidence intervals [CI]) for discrete variables, the Student's t test for normally distributed continuous variables and the Mann-Whitney test for non-normally distributed continuous variables. Kaplan-Meier survival curves were constructed for time-dependent variables and analysed with both the log-rank and the Breslow tests to detect differences in both the number and timing of events. Multiple logistical regression, using entry of variables at a significance level of 0.2 from univariate analysis and stepwise rejection of variables at the 0.05 level of significance, was used to identify independent predictors of death or readmission. All analyses were performed using SPSS for Windows (9.0).

Results

Baseline characteristics

Analysis of the baseline demographic and clinical characteristics of the two groups showed that these were predominantly old and frail patients with significant co-morbidity likely to complicate treatment (see Table 7.1). The age and gender distributions of the two cohorts were almost identical. There were some notable differences between the two groups, however. For example, significantly more Scottish patients lived alone, were admitted with acute pulmonary oedema and were assessed to be dependent for at least one activity of daily living at hospital discharge. Scottish patients were also hospitalized, on average, for two days more

Table 7.1: Baseline demographic and clinical characteristics of Australian and Scottish patients at the time of hospital discharge

	Australia (n = 200)	Scotland (n = 157)
Demographic profile		
Male	120 (60%)	92 (59%)
Mean age in years	76 (8)	75 (8)
Living alone [†]	68 (34%)	72 (46%)
Routine home support services at discharge	90 (45%)	60 (38%)
Heart failure profile		
Previously treated for heart failure [†]	143 (71%)	95 (61%)
Previous admission for heart failure [†]	103 (51%)	69 (44%)
Moderate to severe left ventricular systolic dysfunction	154 (77%)[*]	135 (86%)
Co-morbidity		
Ischaemic heart disease: past myocardial infarction	156 (78%): 141 (70%)	111 (71%): 98 (62%)
Chronic airways disease	71 (36%)	44 (28%)
Chronic hypertension	132 (66%)	90 (57%)
Non-insulin/insulin dependent diabetes [†]	64 (32%)	35 (22%)
Mean Charlson Index of Co-morbidity score [§]	3.1 (1.4)	2.5 (1.2)
Index admission profile		
Median duration of index admission in days [§]	5 (3, 8)	7 (4, 10)
Acute pulmonary oedema [‡]	104 (52%)	107 (68%)
Acute myocardial ischaemia	28 (14%)	32 (20%)
Pharmacotherapy at hospital discharge		
Mean number of prescribed medications [§]	7.6 (2.1)	6.0 (1.9)
Diuretic	193 (96%)	145 (92%)
Long-acting nitrate [§]	148 (74%)	47 (30%)
ACE inhibitor	142 (71%)	120 (76%)
Digoxin [§]	131 (66%)	66 (42%)
Aspirin [§]	147 (73%)	76 (48%)
β-adrenoceptor antagonist [§]	56 (28%)	5 (3%)
Blood profile at hospital discharge		
Sodium mmol/L	138 (3.3)	138 (3.1)
Potassium	4.0 (0.5)	4.3 (0.5)
Creatinine mmol/l [†]	151 (81)	137 (60)
Haemodynamic status at hospital discharge		
Heart rate (beats/minute)	77 (13)	77 (15)
Systolic/diastolic blood pressure (mm Hg)	123 (21) / 67 (11)	121 (20) / 69 (11)
Sinus rhythm: atrial fibrillation (%)	63: 31	73: 25
Status at hospital discharge		
'Dry weight' (kg)	71 (15)	68 (16)
Dependent for ≥ one activity of daily living [‡]	97 (49%)	109 (69%)
NYHA Class II : III : IV (%)	45: 45: 10	57: 36: 7

[†] = < 0.05, [‡] = < 0.01, [§] = < 0.001. Normally distributed and skewed values shown as a mean (SD) and median (IQR).

than their Australian counterparts. Conversely, Australian patients were more likely to come from a non-English-speaking background, and to have been previously treated and hospitalized for chronic heart failure. They also had on average greater renal dysfunction and more co-morbidity overall (for example, chronic angina pectoris and diabetes).

Prescribed pharmacotherapy

Consistent with their greater overall burden of disease, Australian patients were prescribed more extensive pharmacotherapy. However, in both countries most patients were prescribed a diuretic (n = 338), the principal drug of choice in this respect being frusemide (93%) – a median total daily dose of 80 mg was prescribed in both countries. Overall, 36% and 32% Australian and Scottish patients were prescribed what is usually considered a high daily dose of frusemide (> 120 mg).[29]

Although most patients in both countries were prescribed an angiotensin-converting enzyme (ACE) inhibitor, the agents of choice and dosages in which they were prescribed were different. In Scotland the most commonly prescribed agents were enalapril (45%) and lisinopril (32%) in a mean total daily dose of 20 mg and 15 mg respectively. In Australia the most commonly prescribed agents were captopril (40%) and enalapril (35%) in a mean total daily dose of 73 mg and 11 mg respectively. Overall, however, a similar proportion of patients in Australia and Scotland were prescribed what are usually considered to be 'high' doses (75–150 mg captopril, 21–40 mg enalapril/lisinopril or equivalent; 20% vs 18%), 'medium' doses (25–50 mg captopril, 10–20 mg enalapril or lisinopril, or equivalent; 64% vs 66%), or 'low' doses (< 25 mg captopril, < 10 mg enalapril or lisinopril or equivalent; 16% at both centers) of ACE inhibition.[25]

The two cohorts were somewhat different in respect to prescribed long-acting nitrate, digoxin and b-adrenoceptor antagonist therapy, the Adelaide cohort receiving significantly more of these agents. As with ACE inhibitors, however, prescribed dosages were similar when used. For example, the prescribed mean daily dose of digoxin among the Australian and Scottish cohort respectively was 114 mg vs 111 mg.

Health outcomes

Overall, 49% of Scottish patients remained 'event-free' within three months compared with 55% of patients in Australia. Figure 7.1 represents the probability of event-free survival (unplanned readmission or out-of-hospital death) during this period. As such, the two event curves were similar for the two cohorts ($p = 0.76$; log-rank test).

In Australia the 100 'usual care' patients accumulated a total of 30 unplanned readmissions compared with the 43 readmissions accumulated by the 75 'usual care' patients in Scotland ($p < 0.01$). However, a similar proportion of Australian and Scottish patients (15% and 12%, respectively) accumulated ≥ 2 unplanned

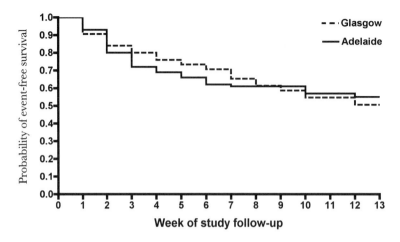

There was no significant difference between groups with respect to the number and timing of events according to the log-rank and Breslow tests.

Figure 7.1: Probability of event-free survival within three months of an acute admission for heart failure in Adelaide, Australia (n =100), and Glasgow, Scotland (n = 75).

readmissions during this period (NS). Therefore, the difference in the total number of unplanned readmissions was caused largely by a small number of Scottish patients being repeatedly readmitted during this period. Despite the disparity in hospital events, there was no significant difference between the two study cohorts in respect to days of hospitalization, with Australian and Scottish patients accumulating a median of 0.6 vs 0.9 days, respectively, of hospitalization/patient/month (NS).

Survival was also similar in the two cohorts, with 19% vs 16% of Scottish and Australian patients dying within three months of discharge, respectively. Figure 7.2 represents the survival curves for the two cohorts, which, like those for event-free survival, are similar ($p = 0.69$; log-rank test).

According to the initial univariate analysis, the following were associated with an increased probability of unplanned readmission or death within three months – greater co-morbidity (higher Charlson Index score[29]), a previous hospitalization for chronic heart failure, hypertension, atrial fibrillation, anaemia, absence of an ACE inhibitor, higher NYHA classification, greater number of prescribed medications, presence of severe renal function impairment and longer length of stay.

On subsequent multivariate analysis, severe renal function impairment, a previous hospitalization for heart failure, longer index hospitalization and a higher Charlson Index of Co-morbidity score were found to be significant independent predictors in this regard (see Table 7.2). Although not retained in the final model, atrial fibrillation was also associated with a strong probability of readmission or death (adjusted OR 2.2, 95% CI 0.92, 5.2; $p = 0.08$).

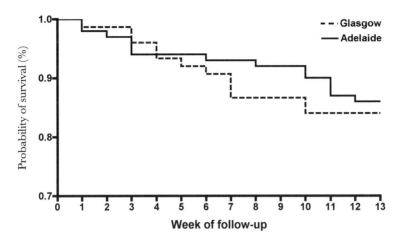

Figure 7.2: Probability of survival within three months of an acute admission for heart failure in Adelaide, Australia (n =100), and Glasgow, Scotland (n = 75).

Table 7.2: Independent correlates of event-free survival within three months of hospital discharge in Australian and Scottish patients with heart failure subject to usual care (n = 175)

Unplanned readmission or out-of-hospital death within three months	No (n = 92)	Yes (n = 83)	p value	Odds ratio (95% CIs)
Severe renal dysfunction	7 (8%)	21 (25%)	0.015	4.4 (1.33, 14)
Previous hospitalization for heart failure	33 (36%)	58 (70%)	0.025	2.3 (1.11, 4.8)
Longer index hospitalization (days) [†]	7.0 (5.1)	8.2 (8.3)	0.048	2.7 (1.01, 7.1)
Higher Charlson Index of Co-morbidity score [‡]	2.6 (1.3)	3.1 (1.4)	0.050	1.3 (1.00, 1.7)

Mean values are presented with SD in brackets. Adjusted odds ratios represent: [†] = 10 or more days of hospitalization and [‡] = each incremental score of one.

Study implications

This study represents the first detailed comparison of the clinical characteristics and health outcomes of older and therefore more representative patients with heart failure requiring acute hospitalization in two different countries. It suggests that patients with heart failure admitted to a tertiary referral hospital servicing an urban population in Glasgow[14], Scotland, are remarkably similar to those admitted to a comparable institution in Adelaide, Australia.[5] Unlike most clinical trials[28], the study cohorts were older and included a large proportion of women. Consistent with previous reports, many patients had at least one non-cardiac condition likely to complicate treatment and to adversely affect their health.

There were some differences in the baseline characteristics and prescribed treatment of the two cohorts. Overall, the Australian cohort had more co-morbidity and had been treated for heart failure over a longer period. Consistent with a recent report of treatment practices among the different countries partici-pating in the PRIME-II[25] and CHARM Study[30], the use of digoxin in Scotland was low compared with that in Australia. However, proportionately more Australian patients were eligible for digoxin therapy[14] because of prior hospitaliza-tion for heart failure. More Australian patients were also prescribed a b-adreno-ceptor antagonist. This, once again, may reflect their more extensive history of heart failure, or because they were treated by cardiologists who have been shown to be more up to date with the current literature and guidelines.[31, 32] Conversely, Scottish patients were, on average, admitted for two days longer than their Australian counterparts during their index hospitalization.

Despite these differences, the health outcomes independently observed in patients with heart failure living in either the southern or northern hemisphere were similar. Although the observed similarities may simply reflect pure serendipity, the observed outcomes are consistent with those emanating from other developed countries. For example, in a comparable study of specialist nurse inter-vention by Rich and colleagues in the United States, the number of reported 'usual care' patients (n = 140) who remained event-free at three months was 54%, 16% needed two or more readmissions and 12% died.[7] Although the mortality was lower in this particular cohort, this most probably reflects the fact that fewer patients with left ventricular systolic dysfunction were recruited, its presence usually being a major determinant of survival[33] but not of morbidity.[11] Moreover, the 6–12 month mortality and morbidity rates observed in these two cohorts (data not shown) are consistent with recent large-scale reports from a number of devel-oped countries (including Scotland) that suggest that about 50% of patients with heart failure are readmitted within 6 months and 33% die within 12 months of acute hospitalization.[34]

Suboptimal use of proven pharmacological agents (particularly ACE inhibitors) is one possible reason for the consistently high morbidity and mortality among patients admitted with heart failure.[35] During the period of study, however, most patients were receiving appropriate pharmacotherapy. The incremental benefits of nurse-led programmes in reducing readmissions and prolonging event-free survival among such patients[5–8] supports the supposition that a multitude of factors, including treatment non-adherence and suboptimal self-care behaviour patterns overall, contribute to consistently high morbidity and mortality.

Pooled multivariate analysis of possible demographic and clinical determinants of event-free survival within three months of hospital discharge suggested that the healthcare system in which the patients were managed had little influence on outcome. Consistent with previous studies, concurrent renal failure (especially when resulting in intolerance to ACE inhibitors)[36, 37], a history of previous admissions for heart failure, extended length of stay and a higher co-morbid burden were all independently associated with a worse health outcome.

Limitations

Any interpretation of these data needs to consider a number of study limitations, including the fact that this was not a prospective study with formal power calculations to determine any observed differences. Despite fairly broad inclusion and minimal exclusion criteria, both studies introduced some selection bias. For example, patients with 'diastolic' left ventricular dysfunction are undoubtedly under-represented. Moreover, both studies selected patients from urban, largely disadvantaged populations admitted to tertiary affiliated hospitals and represent only moderately sized cohorts. Furthermore, we were unable to completely match all baseline and outcome data for univariate and multivariate comparisons.

Conclusions

This study, however, represents the first detailed examination of the characteristics and subsequent health outcomes of patients with chronic heart failure admitted to hospital in two different countries. Although these data need to be confirmed in larger cohorts and in a more systematic way, they suggest that, irrespective of the healthcare system, it is the syndrome of heart failure and the inherent problems it engenders for the individual that largely determine health outcomes.

Summary

In a series of studies we have confirmed that burden of heart failure remains onerous both on an individual and on a population basis. In the absence of effective prevention, the modern healthcare system has to cope with a large number of older patients with heart failure and other disease states likely to complicate treatment. These patients are similar the world over.

We have also shown that a specialist nurse-led intervention in heart failure, especially when incorporating a multidisciplinary approach and home visits, is particularly effective in improving health outcomes among patients with heart failure. As long as it is adapted to the local healthcare environment, this type of management programme represents a cost-effective means to reducing costly admissions for heart failure within the healthcare system, while improving the overall quality of life of individual patients with this truly 'malignant' condition.

References

1. Weinberger M, Oddone EZ, Henderson WG. Does increased access to primary care reduce hospital readmissions? *New Engl J Med* 1996; 334: 1441–7.

2. Mold JW, Stein HF. The cascade effect in clinical care of patients. *N Engl J Med* 1986; 314: 512–14.

3. Rich MW. Heart failure disease management: A critical review. *J Card Fail* 1999; 5: 64–75.

4. Naylor M, Brooten D, Jones R, et al. Comprehensive discharge planning for the hospitalized elderly. *Ann Intern Med* 1994; 120: 999–1006.

5. Naylor MD, Brooten D, Campbell R, et al. Comprehensive discharge planning and home follow-up of hospitalized elders: A randomized clinical trial. *JAMA* 1999; 281: 613-20.

6. Jaarsma T, Halfens R, Huijer Abu-Saad H, et al. Effects of education and support on self-care and resource utilization in patients with heart failure. *Eur Heart J* 1999; 20: 673–82.

7. Rich MW, Beckham V, Wittenberg C, et al. A multidisciplinary intervention to prevent the readmission of elderly patients with congestive heart failure. *New Engl J Med* 1995; 333: 1190–5.

8. Cline C, Israelsson B, Willenheimer R, et al. A cost effective management programme for heart failure reduces hospitalisation. *Heart* 1998; 80: 442–6.

9. Stewart S, Pearson S, Luke CG, et al. Effects of a home based intervention on unplanned readmissions and out-of-hospital deaths. *J Am Geriatr Soc* 1998; 46: 174–80.

10. Stewart S, Pearson S, Horowitz JD. Effects of a home-based intervention among patients with chronic congestive heart failure. *Arch Intern Med* 1998; 158: 1067–72.

11. Stewart S, Vandenbroek A, Pearson S, et al. Prolonged beneficial effects of a home-based intervention on unplanned readmissions and mortality among congestive heart failure patients. *Arch Intern Med* 1999; 159: 257–61.

12. Stewart S, Marley JE, Horowitz JD. Effects of a multidisciplinary, home-based intervention on unplanned readmissions and survival among patients with chronic congestive heart failure: A randomised controlled study. *Lancet* 1999; 354: 1077–83.

13. Blue L, Strong E, Murdoch DR, et al. Improving long-term outcome with specialist nurse intervention in heart failure: A randomised trial. *Eur Heart J* 2000; 21: 151.

14. Blue L, Strong E, Murdoch DR, et al. Randomised controlled trial of specialist nurse intervention in heart failure. *BMJ* 2001; 323: 715–18.

15. Moser DK, Macko MJ, Worster P. Community case management decreases rehospitalisation rates and costs, and improves quality of life in heart failure patients with preserved and non-preserved left ventricular function: A randomised controlled trial. *Circulation* 2000; 102: II 749.

16. Krumholz HM, Amatruda J, Mattera JA, et al. Randomized trial of a nurse-directed educational intervention to prevent readmission of patients with heart failure. *Circulation* 2000; 102: II 749.

17. Riegel BJ, Carlson B, Kopp Z, et al. Is computer-supported telephonic case-management as effective in a Latino heart failure population? *Circulation* 2000; 102: II 749.

18. Doughty RN, Wright SP, Walsh HJ, et al. Randomised, controlled trial of integrated heart failure management: The Auckland Heart Failure Management Study. *Eur Heart J* 2002; 23: 139–46.

19. Kornowski R, Zeeli D, Averbuch M, et al. Intensive home-care surveillance prevents hospitalization and improves morbidity rates among elderly patients with severe congestive heart failure. *Am Heart J* 1995; 129: 162–6.

20.   West J, Miller N, Parker K, et al. A comprehensive management system for heart failure improves clinical outcomes and reduces medical resource utilization. *Am J Cardiol* 1997; 79: 58–63.

21.   Fonarow GC, Stevenson LW, Walden JA, et al. Impact of a comprehensive heart failure management program on hospital readmissions and functional status of patients with advanced heart failure. *J Am Coll Cardiol* 1997; 30: 725–32.

22.   Shah NB, Der E, Ruggerio C, et al. Prevention of hospitalizations for heart failure with an interactive home monitoring program. *Am Heart J* 1998; 135: 373–8.

23.   Stewart S, Blue L (eds). *Improving Outcomes in Chronic Heart Failure with Specialist Nurse Intervention: A Practical Guide.* London: BMJ Publishers, 2000.

24.   Stewart S, Blue L, Capewell S, et al. Poles apart, but are they the same? A comparative study of Australian and Scottish patients with chronic heart failure. *Eur J Heart Fail* 2001; 3: 249–55.

25.   Van Veldhuisen DJ, Charlesworth A, Crijns HJ, et al. Differences in drug treatment of chronic heart failure between European countries. *Eur Heart J* 1999; 20: 666–72.

26.   Massie BM, Cleland JG, Armstrong PW, et al. Regional differences in the characteristics and treatment of patients participating in an international heart failure trial. The Assessment of Treatment with Lisinopril and Survival (ATLAS) Trial Investigators. *J Card Fail* 1998; 4: 3–8.

27.   Bart BA, Ertl G, Held P, et al. Contemporary management of patients with left ventricular systolic dysfunction. Results from the study of patients intolerant of converting enzyme inhibitors (SPICE) registry. *Eur Heart J* 1999; 20: 1182–90.

28.   Petrie M, Berry C, Stewart S, et al. Failing ageing hearts. *Eur Heart J* 2001; 22: 1978–90.

29.   Charlson ME, Pompei P, Ales KL, et al. A new method of classifying prognostic co-morbidity in longitudinal studies: development and validation. *J Chronic Dis* 1987; 40: 373–83.

30.   McMurray JJ for the CHARM Investigators. Is the United Kingdom the least evidence-based country in the world for the treatment of chronic heart failure? *Heart* 2000; 83: S52.

31.   Stafford RS, Saglam D, Blumenthal D. National patterns of angiotensin-converting enzyme inhibitor use in congestive heart failure. *Arch Intern Med* 1997; 157: 2460–4.

32.   Edep ME, Shah NB, Tateo IM, et al. Difference between primary care physicians and cardiologists in management of congestive heart failure: Relation to practice guidelines. *J Am Coll Cardiol* 1997; 30: 518–26.

33.   Vasan RS, Larson RG, Benjamin EJ, et al. Congestive heart failure in subjects with normal versus reduced left ventricular ejection fraction. *J Am Coll Cardiol* 1999; 33: 1948–55.

34.   Stewart S, MacIntyre K, McCleod MC, et al. Trends in heart failure hospitalisations in Scotland, 1990–1996: An epidemic that has reached its peak? *Eur Heart J* 2000; 22: 209–17.

35.   Luzier A, Forrest A, Adelman M, et al. Impact of angiotensin-converting enzyme inhibitor underdosing on rehospitalization rates in congestive heart failure. *Am J Cardiol* 1998; 82: 465–9.

36.   MacDowall P, Kaira P, O'Donoghue D, et al. Risk of morbidity from renovascular disease in elderly patients with congestive cardiac failure. *Lancet* 1998; 352: 13–16.

37.   Krumholz HM, Chen YT, Bradford WD, et al. Variations in and correlates of length of stay in academic hospitals among patients with heart failure resulting from systolic dysfunction. *Am J Manag Care* 1999; 5: 715–23.

Publications arising from this research

Cost benefits of a nurse-led intervention in chronic heart failure

Stewart S, Davey M, De-Sanctis M, March G, Hooper J, Pearson J, Luke CG. Home medication management: A study of patients post-hospitalisation. *Australian Pharmacist* 1995; 4: 472–6.

Stewart S, Pearson S, Luke CG, Horowitz JD. Effects of a home-based intervention on unplanned readmissions and out-of-hospital deaths. *Journal of the American Geriatric Society* 1998; 46: 174–80.

Rubenstein LZ, Stewart S, Scholl M, Bernabei R, Bula C, Jones D, Wieland D. In-home programs of prevention and comprehensive geriatric assessment: international perspectives. *The Australasian Journal of Ageing* 1998; 17: S73–S78.

Stewart S, Pearson S, Horowitz JD. Effects of a home-based intervention among congestive heart failure patients discharged from acute hospital care. *Archives of Internal Medicine* 1998; 158: 1067–72.

McMurray JJV, Stewart S. Nurse-led multidisciplinary intervention in chronic heart failure. (Editorial) *Heart* 1998; 80: 430–1.

Stewart S, Vandenbroek AJ, Pearson S, Horowitz JD. Prolonged beneficial effects of a home-based intervention on unplanned readmissions and mortality among congestive heart failure patients. *Archives of Internal Medicine* 1999; 159: 257–61.

Stewart S, Pearson S. Uncovering a multitude of sins: Medication management in the home post acute hospitalisation among the chronically ill. *Australian and New Zealand Journal of Medicine* 1999; 29: 220–7.

Pearson S, Stewart S, Rubenach S. Is health-related quality of life among older, chronically ill patients associated with unplanned readmission to hospital? *Australian and New Zealand Journal of Medicine* 1999; 29: 701–6.

Stewart S, Marley JE, Horowitz JD. Effects of a multidisciplinary, home-based intervention on unplanned readmissions and survival among patients with congestive heart failure: A randomised controlled study. *The Lancet* 1999; 354: 1077–83.

Stewart S, Blue L, Capewell S, Horowitz JD, McMurray JJV. Poles apart, but are they the same? A comparative study of Australian and Scottish patients with chronic heart failure. *European Journal of Heart Failure* 2001; 3: 249–55.

Davidson P, Stewart S, Elliott D, Daly J, Cockburn J. Addressing the burden of heart failure in Australia: the scope for home based interventions. *Journal of Cardiovascular Nursing* 2001; 16: 56–68.

Stewart S, Horowitz JD. Detecting early clinical deterioration in chronic heart failure patients post acute hospitalisation – A critical component of multidisciplinary, home-based intervention? *European Journal of Heart Failure* 2002; 4: 345–51.

Stewart S, Blue L, Walker A, *et al.* An economic analysis of specialist heart failure management in the United Kingdom – Can we afford not to implement it? *European Heart Journal* – In press.

Epidemiology and cost of heart failure

MacIntyre K, Capewell S, Stewart S, *et al.* Evidence of improving prognosis in heart failure: Trends in case-fatality in 66,547 patients hospitalised between 1986 and 1995. *Circulation* 2000; 102: 1126–31.

Stewart S, MacIntyre K, McCleod MC, Bailey AE, McMurray JJV. Trends in heart failure hospitalisations in Scotland, 1990–1996: An epidemic that has reached its peak? *European Heart Journal* 2000; 22: 209–17.

McMurray JJV, Stewart S. Epidemiology, aetiology and prognosis of heart failure. *Heart* 2000; 83: 596–602.

Stewart S, MacIntyre K, Hole DA, Capewell S, McMurray JJV. More malignant than cancer? Five-year survival following a first admission for heart failure in Scotland? *European Journal of Heart Failure* 2001; 3: 315–22.

Horowitz JD, Stewart S. Heart failure in the elderly – the epidemic we had to have? (Editorial). *Medical Journal of Australia* 2001; 174: 432–3.

MacIntyre K, Stewart S, McMurray JJV. Is prognosis improving in heart failure? Cardiology *Review* 2001; 18: 29–35.

Stewart S, McMurray JJV. Heart failure patients – older and more complicated: An increasing challenge to the health care system! *Coronary Health Care* 2001; 5: 121–5.

Stewart S, Jenkins A, Buchan S, Capewell S, McGuire A, McMurray JJV. The current cost of heart failure in the UK – An economic analysis. *European Journal of Heart Failure* 2002; 4: 361–71.

Stewart S, Demers C, Murdoch DR, *et al.* Substantial between hospital variation in outcome following acute admission with heart failure. *European Heart Journal* 2002; 23: 650–57.

Stewart S, MacIntyre K, McMurray JJV. Heart failure in a cold climate: seasonal variation in heart failure-related morbidity and mortality. *Journal of American College of Cardiology* 2002; 39: 760–66.

Stewart S, MacIntyre K, Capewell S, McMurray JJV. An ageing population and heart failure: An increasing burden in the 21st Century? *Heart* – In press.

McMurray JJV, Stewart S. The burden of heart failure. *European Heart Journal* 2002; 4: D50–D58.

Index